T0212174

Lecture Notes of the Institute for Computer Sciences, Social Informatics and Telecommunications Engineering 393

More information about this series at http://www.springer.com/series/8197

José Antonio Marmolejo-Saucedo ·
Pandian Vasant · Igor Litvinchev ·
Roman Rodríguez-Aguilar ·
Jania Astrid Saucedo-Martínez (Eds.)

Computer Science and Engineering in Health Services

5th EAI International Conference, COMPSE 2021
Virtual Event, July 29, 2021
Proceedings

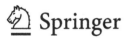
Springer

Editors
José Antonio Marmolejo-Saucedo🄳
Panamerican University
Mexico, Distrito Federal, Mexico

Pandian Vasant
Universiti Teknologi Petronas
Tronoh, Perak, Malaysia

Igor Litvinchev🄳
Universidad Autónoma de Nuevo León
San Nicolás de los Garza, Mexico

Roman Rodríguez-Aguilar🄳
Panamerican University
Mexico, Mexico

Jania Astrid Saucedo-Martínez🄳
Universidad Autónoma de Nuevo León
San Nicolás de los Garza, Mexico

ISSN 1867-8211   ISSN 1867-822X (electronic)
Lecture Notes of the Institute for Computer Sciences, Social Informatics
and Telecommunications Engineering
ISBN 978-3-030-87494-0   ISBN 978-3-030-87495-7 (eBook)
https://doi.org/10.1007/978-3-030-87495-7

This Springer imprint is published by the registered company Springer Nature Switzerland AG
The registered company address is: Gewerbestrasse 11, 6330 Cham, Switzerland

Preface

We are pleased to introduce the proceedings of our 5th edition of the EAI International Conference on Computer Science and Engineering in Health Services (COMPSE 2021) which took place on July 29, 2021, in Mexico City. In these difficult times, the conference brought together many researchers, practitioners, and experts whose outstanding contributions continue to increase our knowledge in different fields. For the second year, we embrace the great changes and challenges in our daily lives due to the COVID-19 pandemic by taking advantage of technology and all the necessary tools to bring this virtual conference and its remarkable works to all the scientific and academic communities

The complexity of real-life problems remains to be addressed in this forum seeking the development of knowledge related to topics of great importance worldwide. The following tracks build the framework of this conference: Track 1, the Application of Tools Delivered by the COVID-19; Track 2, Health Services; Track 3 Computer and Data Science; and Track 4, Industry 4.0 in Logistics and Supply Chain.

The technical program of this annual edition consisted of 17 full papers which contain remarkable research that will certainly encourage participants and many others to continue this important work in the future. A special workshop was also held this year on machine learning and data mining: applications in economics and business science.

The 2021 Steering Committee was integrated by Prof. Imrich Chlamtac (University of Trento, Italy), and Prof. Igor Litvinchev (Universidad Autónoma de Nuevo León, Mexico), whose coordination was essential to the success of this virtual conference. Prof. Roman Rodriguez Aguilar (Universidad Panamericana, Mexico) and Prof. Jania Astrid Martinez Saucedo (Universidad Autónoma de Nuevo León), members of the Organization Committee, also contributed to the thoroughly executed logistics. The Technical Program Committee, led by Prof. Tomas Salais (Universidad Autónoma de Nuevo León, Mexico), Prof. Tatiana Romanova (National Academy of Science, Ukraine), Prof. Utku Kose (Demirel University, Turkey), Prof. Pandiant Vasant (Universiti Teknologi, Malaysia), and Prof. Igor Litvinchev (Universidad Autónoma de Nuevo León, Mexico), did an excellent job in achieving a high-quality cutting-edge content for this year. In this edition, COMPSE 2021 had the participation of Prof. José Antonio Marmolejo from the Universidad Panamericana México as keynote in the plenary conference. The title of the plenary was "Design and Development of Digital Twins in Business: A Prospective Vision".

Many thanks and all our respect go to Natasha Onefrei, Conference Manager, for all her support and our sincere appreciation goes to all authors who submitted their work for the edition of this year. Lastly, we thank the Panamerican University in Mexico for its great efforts in making this conference possible and the thorough work to successfully achieve terrific results of this 5th edition of EAI COMPSE 2021.

August 2021   Jania Astrid Saucedo-Martínez

Organization

Steering Committee

Imrich Chlamtac   University of Trento, Italy
Igor Litvinchev   Universidad Autónoma de Nuevo León, Mexico

Organizing Committee

General Chairs

Roman Rodriguez Aguilar   Universidad Panamericana, Mexico
Jania Astrid Saucedo   Universidad Autónoma de Nuevo León, Mexico
   Martínez

Technical Program Committee Chairs

Tomas Salais   Universidad Autónoma de Nuevo León, Mexico
Tatiana Romanova   National Academy of Sciences, Ukraine
Utku Kose   Demirel University, Turkey
Pandiant Vasant   Universiti Teknologi PETRONAS, Malaysia
Igor Litvinchev   Universidad Autónoma de Nuevo León, Mexico

Sponsorship and Exhibit Chair

Antonia Paola Salgado   Universidad Panamericana, Mexico
   Reyes

Local Chair

Eulalio González Anta   Universidad Panamericana, Mexico

Workshops Chair

Johanna Bolaños   Universidad Autónoma de Nuevo León, Mexico

Publicity and Social Media Chair

Johanna Bolaños   Universidad Autónoma de Nuevo León, Mexico
Carlos Regalao Noriega   Universidad Simón Bolívar, Colombia

Publications Chair

Jania Astrid Saucedo   Universidad Autónoma de Nuevo León, Mexico
  Martínez

Web Chair

Johanna Bolaños   Universidad Autónoma de Nuevo León, Mexico

Technical Program Committee

Deniz Ozdemir   Solvoyo, Turkey
Alexander De Jesus Pulido   Universidad Simón Bolívar, Colombia
  Rojano
Omer Deperlioglu   Afyon Kocatepe University, Turkey
Olympia Roeva   Institute of Biophysics and Biomedical Engineering,
                                  Bulgaria
Steed Huang   Carleton University, Canada
Dadmehr Rahbari   University of Qom, Ira
Thanatchai   Suranaree University of Technology, Thailand
  Kulworawanichpong
Abdellah Derghal   LGEA Laboratory, Algeria
Ana Carolina   National University of Austral Patagonia, Argentina
Bharat Singh   Nomad Digital GMBH, Germany
Dieu N. Vo   Ho Chi Minh City University of Technology, Vietnam
Emilio Jimenez   University of La Rioja, Spain
Goran Klepac   Hrvatski Telekom, Croatia
John Escobar   Pontificia Universidad Javeriana, Cali, Colombia
Jorge Luis Rojas Arce   Universidad Nacional Autónoma de México, Mexico
Mario Pavone   University of Catania, Italy
Monika Chris   Frequentis AG Austria, Romania
Nuno Pombo   University of Beira Interior, Portugal
Raquel Joao Fonseca   Universidade de Lisboa, Portugal
Rosana Cavalcante de   Brazilian Agricultural Research Corporation, Brazil
  Oliveira
Rustem Popa   "Dunarea de Jos" University in Galati, Romania
Ugo Fiore   University of Naples Federico II, Italy
Vipul Sharma   DAV University, India
Warusia Yassin   Universiti Teknikal Malaysia Melaka, Malaysia
Wei Siang Hoh   Universiti Malaysia Perlis, Malaysia
Bhupesh Singh   G. B. Pant University of Agriculture and Technology,
                                  India

Contents

Application of Tools Derived from Covid

Tool Development for the Optimal Supply of Medical Oxygen Delivered
at Home.. 3
    Cristina De-los-Santos Ventura and Jania Astrid Saucedo Martínez

A Life Cycle Assessment (LCA) of Antibacterial Gel Production 12
    Valeria Enríquez-Martínez, Isabel J. Niembro-García,
    and José A. Marmolejo-Saucedo

An Alternative Model to Estimate Annual Budget Through TDABC
Methodology in Hospitals 28
    José Luis Hernández Arredondo, Elí Gerardo Zorrilla Uribe,
    and Zaida Estafanía Alarcón Bernal

ARM: A Real-Time Health Monitoring Mobile Application 45
    Saeid Pourroostaei Ardakani, Xuting Wu, Shuning Pan, and Xinyu Gao

Computer and Data Science

Network Coding and Dispersal Information with TCP
for Content Delivery 63
    Francisco de Asís López-Fuentes, Raúl Antonio Ortega-Vallejo,
    and Ricardo Marcelín-Jiménez

Sentiment Analysis Model on Twitter About Video Streaming Platforms
in Mexico 73
    Rosalia Andrade-Gonzalez and Roman Rodriguez-Aguilar

An Asset Index Proposal for Households in Mexico Applying the Mixed
Principal Components Analysis Methodology 88
    Lorena DelaTorre-Díaz and Román Rodriguez-Aguilar

Health Systems

A Data-Driven Study to Highlight the Correlations Between Ambient
Factors and Emotion 109
    Saeid Pourroostaei Ardakani, Xinyang Liu, and Hongcheng Xie

Telerehabilitation Prototype for Postural Disorder Monitoring
in Parkinson Disease   129
   Jorge L. Rojas-Arce, Luis Jimenez-Angeles,
   and Jose Antonio Marmolejo-Saucedo

Analysis of Medical Tourism and the Effect of Using Digital Tools
to Profile Travelers in Mexico   143
   Edmundo Arrioja-Castrejón and Andrée Marie López-Fernández

Performance Evaluation of Healthcare Systems Using Data
Envelopment Analysis   162
   Itzel Viridiana González-Badillo and Zaida Estefanía Alarcón-Bernal

Industry 4.0 in Logistics and Supply Chain

Organizational Efficiency in the Implementation of 4.0 Technologies
in Logistics Operators in the Colombian Caribbean Region   177
   Jania Astrid Saucedo-Martinez, Carlos Jose Regalao-Noriega,
   and Luis Ortiz-Ospino

Sustainability Model for the Livestock Sector in the Department
of La Guajira - Colombia.   196
   Helia Rosa del Carmen Daza Guerra, Carlos Jose Regalao-Noriega,
   and Karen Acosta Triana

Design of a Logistics Network Using Analytical Techniques
and Agent-Based Simulation.   216
   Jose Antonio Marmolejo-Saucedo, Roman Rodriguez-Aguilar,
   Gerardo Meza Callejas, Mitchell Santiago Kelley Urbieta,
   Saul Fernando Peregrina Acasuso, and Juan Pablo Gutierrez Girault

A Predictive Performance Measurement System for Decision Making
in the Supply Chain   225
   Loraine Sanchez-Jimenez and Tomás E. Salais-Fierro

Implementation of Intelligent Automation of Production Processes
in the Company Espumados del Litoral in the City of Barranquilla   245
   Estephany Reyes, Jesus Retamozo, Zaida Oliveros, Laura Sierra,
   Jaider Vanegas, and Carlos Jose Regalao-Noriega

A Look at the Literature Review of the Impact of Industry 4.0 on the
Logistics Processes of the Food Sector in Barranquilla.   252
   Carolina Rangel, Jose Otero, Frency Antequera, Yuliana Bonadiez,
   Mary Riquett, and Carlos Jose Regalao-Noriega

Author Index   259

Application of Tools Derived from Covid

Tool Development for the Optimal Supply of Medical Oxygen Delivered at Home

Cristina De-los-Santos Ventura$^{(\boxtimes)}$ and Jania Astrid Saucedo Martínez

Facultad de Ingeniería Mecánica y Eléctrica, Universidad Autónoma de Nuevo León,
Ciudad Universitaria, San Nicolás de los Garza, Nuevo León, Mexico
{cristina.dev,jania.saucedomrt}@uanl.edu.mx

Abstract. Due to the increase in demand for medical oxygen, there is a need to improve the oxygen home delivery service. In this project, we will work with the data of a company specialized in the management of medicinal gases, which has a group of patients who receive medicinal oxygen through cylinders. The goal is to develop a tool that automates the assignment of the optimal distribution center to each patient's zip code, taking into account the distance, supply capacity, and delivery time.

Keywords: Assignment problem · Medical oxygen · Optimization

1 Introduction

Medical oxygen is a gas used for patients who need oxygen therapy. This therapeutic measure has been shown to increase survival in patients with chronic obstructive pulmonary disease (COPD) and respiratory failure, COVID-19, cystic fibrosis, severe asthma attack, pneumonia, etc. [7].

The proper choice of oxygen source depends on many factors, including the amount of oxygen required by the patient; the infrastructure, cost, convenience, patient adaptability, capacity, distribution, and supply chain available for the local production and delivery of medicinal gases; the reliability of the electricity supply; and access to maintenance services and spare parts, etc. [7,9].

Common sources of oxygen are liquid oxygen and oxygen generating plants in bulk storage tanks and oxygen concentrators. The most common source of oxygen storage used in healthcare settings is a cylinder (tank) containing compressed oxygen [9], which can be of different dimensions depending on the patient's need.

Therefore, guarantee the delivery of this gas on time is of utmost importance for the well-being of the patients, which at the same time translates into greater eligibility, trust, and permanence of the clients in the company.

Beca Nacional CONACYT 1009343 and the project Distribution process improvements, PAIYCT CE1803-2.

J. A. Marmolejo-Saucedo et al. (Eds.): COMPSE 2021, LNICST 393, pp. 3–11, 2021.
https://doi.org/10.1007/978-3-030-87495-7_1

1.1   Optimization of Medical Oxygen Cylinder Deliveries

Due to the precise, delicate, and accurate service guarantee in the supply and delivery of medical oxygen cylinders, planning, and logistics distribution represents a key factor in this market. The interaction of transportation in the supply and distribution programs constitutes a dynamic process that requires high coordination.

Without taking into account that the timely delivery of oxygen guarantees customer loyalty and a high level of confidence in the service of their home delivery. Being able to derive an increase in capacity by having a better organization, allowing greater sales, and reducing costs [5].

In the same way, proper management of the supply chain is important since the availability of oxygen must be ensured when the user requires it and even anticipated. In this way, the growing market for this type of services will increase, , since the existence expectancy of a heightened incidence of chronic respiratory diseases, together with the augmentation on the demand for home health care [6].

Thats why a proper assignation of the distribution center to the patients is essential to increase the quality of the delivery service.

1.2   Generalized Assignation Problem, GAP

The classic assignment problem (AP) consists in that given two sets of tasks and agents, assign one agent-to-one task, minimizing costs or maximizing profits [1]. Instead the generalized assignment problem (GAP) each task is assigned to one agent, as in the classic AP, but it allows for the possibility that an agent may be assigned to more than one task, while recognizing that a task may use only part of an agent's capacity rather than all of it [2,3].

GAP has many real-life applications, like a subproblem in routing problem, resource scheduling, scheduling of project networks, storage space allocation, scheduling of payments, assignment jobs to computers, assignment ships to overhaul, fleets of aircraft to trips, or the assignment of school buses to routes [11–13].

However, in most practical applications, each agent requires a quantity of some limited resource to process a given job. Therefore, the assignments have to be made taking into account the resource availability of each agent. The GAP is in practice even more difficult, since most of its applications have a stochastic nature [13].

Stochasticity can be due to two different sources. On the one hand, it appears when the actual capacity of the agents or the amount of resource needed to process the jobs is not known in advance [13].

The second source of stochasticity is uncertainty about the presence or absence of individual jobs. In such cases, there is a set of potential jobs, but only a subset of them will have to be processed. This subset is not known when the assignment has to be decided. e.g. the case of emergency services [13].

The general formulation of the problem is:

$$min \sum_{i} \sum_{j} c_{ij} x_{ij} \tag{1}$$

$$s.t. \sum_{j} a_{ij} x_{ij} \leq b_i \qquad \forall i \in I \tag{2}$$

$$\sum_{i} x_{ij} = 1 \qquad \forall j \in J \tag{3}$$

$$x_{ij} = \{0, 1\} \qquad \forall i \in I, \forall j \in J \tag{4}$$

where c_{ij} is the cost assigning job j to agent i, a_{ij} is the capacity absorption when job j is assigned to agent i, b_i the available capacity of agent i. The assignment variable x_{ij} equals 1 if agent i is to perform job j, 0 otherwise.

The objective function (1) is to minimize the total assignment cost of jobs (j) to agents (i). Constraints (2) designate the capacity availability restriction of each agent. Constraints (3) ensure that each job is assigned to exactly one agentand. Finally, constraints (4) are the condition on the decision variables.

2   Problem Description

In this article a company specialized in industrial and medical gases is studied. Nowadays, this company counts 32 DC in all Mexican Republic (Fig. 1), which only deliver medical oxygen to homecare patients

Of all the DCs, only nine will be analyzed, currently each of these DCs has a group of patients that they visit periodically. For this research, the locations of the patients' zip codes will be taken as the delivery points.

Historically, in this company, the assignments of DCs to each patient have been made manually and with no mathematical background, so not in all cases the closest DC is assigned to the customers, causing a delay in delivery, greater distance traveled and therefore, it makes the service less profitable to the company.

In this case, not vehicular routes will be proposed. Hence, the scope of the project is both the optimal assignation of DC to the patient and, in the future the generation of a schedule of visiting days (according to the distance between a group of patients assigned to a DC, vehicle capacity, and the area in which the client/patient belong).

A generalized assignment problem is proposed, where the objective function is to minimize the distance between the DC and the patient, where a distribution center i can serve n patients j (which in this case are located by ZIP code), and a patient can only be served by one distribution center. And also each DC has a maximum number of patients that can attend (zip codes).

These types of problems had been described in different papers, however, each of them had different application purposes. Table 1 gives some examples.

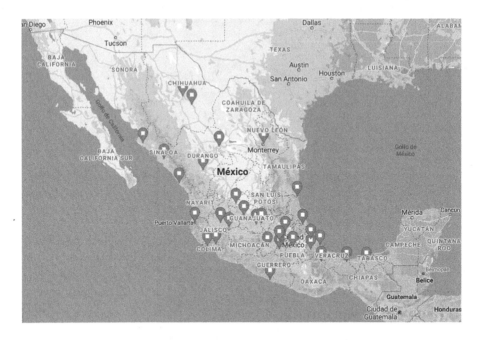

Fig. 1. Locations of distribution centers

Table 1. Literature review

Author	Characteristic
Qian X, 2017 [14]	The Taxi group ride (TGR) is one popular case of taxi ride sharing, where passenger trips with nearby origins and destinations and similar departure times are grouped into a single ride. This study investigates the optimal assignment of a set of passengers for the sake of maximizing total saved travel miles
Albareda-Sambola, 2006 [13]	This paper deals with a stochastic Generalized Assignment Problem with recourse. An assignment of each job to an agent is decided a-priori, and once the subset of jobs that have to be executed is now, reassignments can be performed if there are overloaded agents
Öncan, T., 2007 [12]	In this survey, it was concentrated on real-life applications in scheduling, timetabling, telecommunication, facility location, transportation, production planning, etc. Where Generalized Assignment Problem (GAP) is used to find the optimum assignment of each item to exactly one knapsack, without exceeding the capacity of any knapsack

3 Methodology

3.1 Data Collection

To obtain the exact location of all the national zip codes, it was necessary to use the data from Correos de México, which through treatment in MapInfo [15] software it was able to calculate the centroids of each zip code, these locations (longitude, latitude) were used as a reference of the patients found in that area. The quantity and location of the distribution centers and their location were data provided by the company, also the preference of which DC will be analyzed were made by their requirement.

3.2 Geodesic Distance

For the matrix of distance data, the Geodesic distance formula was used to measure the distance d_{ij}) between the distribution center and every zip code. This formula has been used to generate assignments, which don't necessarily have to have high accuracy concerning the distance between two points, as well as the lack of data on the distances of roads between the different points [10].

$$d_{ij} = \cos^{-1}(b * d * + \cos b * \cos d * \cos(c - a)) * R \tag{5}$$

where: (a, b) and (c, d) represent the pair of longitude and latitude in radians of location i and j, respectively, and R the average radius of Earth.

3.3 Distribution Center Assignation

Being the objective to minimize the distance between the distribution center and the centroids of the ZIP code. Our formulation uses binary variables x_{ij} for each arc (i, j) to denote whether or not the distribution center i is assigned to the zip code j.

$$min \sum_i \sum_j d_{ij} x_{ij} \tag{6}$$

The constraints were defined by: One Zip code just can be attended by one distribution center.

$$\sum_i x_{ij} = 1 \qquad \forall i \in I \tag{7}$$

Also, every DC has a zip code limit assignation (L).

$$\sum_j l_{ij} x_{ij} \leq b_i \qquad \forall j \in J \tag{8}$$

Finally, the constraints enforce the integrality condition on the decision variables.

$$x_{ij} \in \{0, 1\} \qquad \forall i \in I, \forall j \in J \tag{9}$$

3.4   Python as a Programming Tool

To solve the GAP, Python was used as the programming tool to achieve the assignation of the optimal DC to each patient zip code, and it was used the Cplex method to achieve the purpose of this optimization problem.

4   Results

So far, the optimal distribution centers for every patient's zip code were obtained using only distance and a maximum quantity of zip codes that a DC could attend. Comparing the assignments that the company previously used, it was found that 10% of the assignments made by the company were not optimal.

At the same time, it was observed that the decisions being made for assignments was based on the coincidence of whether or not they were within the same State, which caused that the zip codes that were in the outskirts between two DC delivery areas were not attended necessarily by the closest one, these can be seen in Fig. 2. Where it is quite evident that there are better DC options that could serve patients who are in the State of Puebla but who should not necessarily be attended by the DC belonging to that same State.

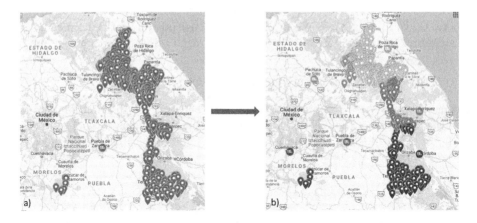

Fig. 2. a) Assignment made for the state of Puebla on its border zip codes that don't belong to their optimal DC , b) The new assignation proposed by the GAP implementation

By distance, it is convenient to change the current patients who belong to the DC of Puebla to the 3 DCs that belong to the state of Veracruz, as well as a DC from the state of Pachuca and another from the state of Morelos, where there would be a saving of 383 km traveled.

This problem can also be observed in the state of Jalisco, where likewise most of the patients on the outskirts of the city of Guadalajara and other nearby towns of the state of Jalisco were assigned to the DC of Guadalajara.

However, due to optimality, these patients should be attended by the DCs of Puerto Vallarta and Ocotlan that belong to the same state, as well as the DCs that are in different states such as Durango, Aguascalientes, Guanajuato and Colima, having a saving of 548 km traveled for the delivery of oxygen cylinders Fig. 3.

In these cases, it was observed that it is due to the fact the patients who belong to the two States mentioned before, are on the outskirts or limits of the urban area, they are adjacent to other states, which causes that they haven't had a correct DC assignment from the beginning.

This phenomenon occurs in most of the non-urban areas of the other states that were analyzed. For the patients that belong to nine states that were analyzed, previously they were served by 15 DCs, however, after applying the GAP it was concluded that it is necessary to include 5 extras DCs to better distribute the workload.

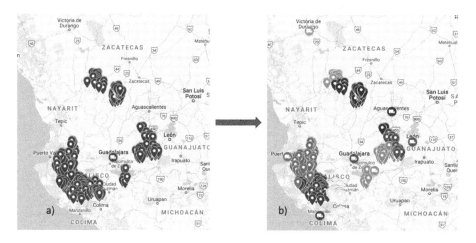

Fig. 3. a) Assignment made for the state of Jalisco on its border zip codes that don't belong to their optimal DC, b) The new assignation proposed by the GAP implementation

An analysis was carried out by States, to determine the savings in distance traveled from the changes that were made when replacing the DC used previously by those that the GAP grants as optimal (Table 2).

Carrying out these changes did not cause any DC to be over-saturated with zip codes to serve, since DCs, have a significant slack for the maximum limits of delivery areas. Although these results still do not translate into monetary savings, it is assumed that the 1,830 km of savings in distance traveled will positively impact the earnings for the home delivery service.

Table 2. Savings on travel distance to deliver medical oxygen at the patients zip codes ubication.

Patient state	DC company assignation	DC GAP assignation	Distance savings (Km)
Colima	Colima, Colima	Puerto Vallarta, Jalisco	128
Guanajuato	Celaya, Guanajuato	Leon, Guanajuato	50
Guanajuato	Celaya, Guanajuato	Queretaro, Queretaro	45
Guanajuato	Celaya, Guanajuato	Ocotlan, Jalisco	50
Hidalgo	Pachuca, Hidalgo	Queretato, Queretaro	50
Hidalgo	Pachuca, Hidalgo	Poza Rica, Veracruz	45
Jalisco	Guadalajara, Jalisco	Durango, Durango	52
Jalisco	Guadalajara, Jalisco	Aguascalientes, Aguascalientes	58
Jalisco	Guadalajara, Jalisco	Leon, Guanajuato	48
Jalisco	Guadalajara, Jalisco	Manzanillo, Colima	165
Jalisco	Guadalajara, Jalisco	Puerto Vallarta, Jalisco	65
Jalisco	Guadalajara, Jalisco	Colima, Colima	90
Jalisco	Guadalajara, Jalisco	Ocotla, Jalisco	70
Puebla	Puebla, Puebla	Cuernavaca, Morelos	38
Puebla	Puebla, Puebla	Pachuca, Hidalgo	70
Puebla	Puebla, Puebla	Cordoba, Veracruz	70
Puebla	Puebla, Puebla	Xalapa, Veracruz	65
Puebla	Puebla, Puebla	Poza Rica, Veracruz	140
Oaxaxa	Oaxaca, Oaxaca	—	0
Sinaloa	Mazatlán	Culiacan, Sinaloa	160
Tabasco	Villa Hermosa, Tabasco	Coatzacoalcos, Veracruz	60
Veracruz	Poza Rica, Veracruz	Xalapa, Veracruz	70
Veracruz	Coatzacoalcos, Veracruz	Cordoba, Veracruz	200
Veracruz	Coatzacoalcos, Veracruz	Tuxtepec, Veracruz	41

5 Conclusions

It was found that there are indeed errors in the manual allocation carried out in the company, so generating a method of choosing the closest distribution center will generate greater benefits in time and savings, by reducing the distances traveled from the distribution center to customers.

However, the project is in the first phase of its development since it's also desired to propose a scheduling scheme for the delivery of medicinal oxygen.

Although, routes will not be proposed, it is necessary to do a territory analysis to assign the days of visit for clients depending on the area in which they reside, and therefore generate savings in the delivery of the product, as well, ensuring the days of visit and at the same time generate reliability in the patients towards the company.

References

1. Litviench, I., Rangel, S., Saucedo, J.: A Lagrangian bound for many-to-many assignment problem. J. Comb. Optim. **19**, 241–257 (2010). https://doi.org/10.1007/s10878-008-9196-3
2. Martello, S., Toth, P.: Knapsack Problems: Algorithms and Computer Implementations. Wiley, New York (1990)
3. Pentico, D.W.: Assignment problems: a golden anniversary survey. Eur. J. Oper. Res. **176**, 774–793 (2007)
4. Chenghua, S., Tonglei, L., Yu, B., Fei, Z.: A heuristics-based parthenogenetic algorithm for he VRP with potential demands and time windows. In: Scientific Programming 2016 (2016)
5. Costantino, F., Di Gravio, G., Tronci, M.: Simulation model of the logistic distribution in a medical oxygen supply chain. In: 19th European Conference on Modelling and Simulation (2005)
6. Grand View Research.: Oxygen Therapy Market Size, Share Global Industry Report 2018–2024. https://www.grandviewresearch.com/industry-analysis/oxygen-therapy-market. Accessed 15 Sept 2020
7. Ortega Ruiz, F., et al.: Continuous home oxygen therapy. Arch. Bronconeumol. **50**(5), 185–200 (2014)
8. Ranieri, L., Digiesi, S., Silvestri, B., Roccotelli, M.: A review of last mile logistics innovations in an externalities cost reduction vision. Sustainability **10**(785), 782 (2018)
9. World Health Organization.: Oxygen sources and distribution for COVID-19 treatment centres: interim guidance. https://apps.who.int/iris/handle/10665/331746?locale-attribute=es&. Accessed 15 Sept 2020
10. Hu, Y., Wang, C., Li, R., Wang, F.: Estimating a large drive time matrix between ZIP codes in the United States: a differential sampling approach. J. Transp. Geogr. **86**, 102770 (2020)
11. Cattrysse, D.G., Van Wassenhove, L.N.: EA survey of algorithms for the generalized assignment problem. Eur. J. Oper. Res. **60**(3), 260–272 (1992). https://doi.org/10.1016/0377-2217(92)90077
12. Öncan, T.: A survey of the generalized assignment problem and its applications. INFOR: Inf. Syst. Oper. Res. **45**(3), 123–141 (2007). https://doi.org/10.3138/infor.45.3.123
13. Albareda-Sambola, M., van der Vlerk, M.H., Fernández, E.: Exact solutions to a class of stochastic generalized assignment problems. Eur. J. Oper. Res. **173**(2), 465–487 (2006). https://doi.org/10.1016/j.ejor.2005.01.035
14. Qian, X., Zhang, W., Ukkusuri, S.V., Yang, C.: Optimal assignment and incentive design in the taxi group ride problem. Transp. Res. Part B: Methodol. **103**, 208–226 (2017). https://doi.org/10.1016/j.trb.2017.03.001
15. MAPINFO. http://www.geobis.com/es/mapinfo-gis-software/. Accessed 10 June 2021

A Life Cycle Assessment (LCA) of Antibacterial Gel Production

Valeria Enríquez-Martínez(✉), Isabel J. Niembro-García,
and José A. Marmolejo-Saucedo

Universidad Panamericana, Facultad de Ingeniería, Augusto Rodin 498,
03920 Ciudad de México, México
{0183164,iniembro,jmarmolejo}@up.edu.mx

Abstract. During the COVID-19 pandemic the antibacterial gel become an important prevention measures to stop the spread of the virus. In Mexico, the demand for preventive hygiene products and health supplies increased more than 50% at the beginning of the pandemic. With the concern of knowing the negative impacts that the high demands of this product can cause to the environment, we took on the task of looking for life cycle assessment (LCA) studies related to the production of antibacterial gel, it was unexpected not to find any scientific information reported about the subject. This paper takes as one of its main motivation the lack of information to accomplish an LCA which is used to evaluate the negative environmental impacts associated with the products or services. The aim of this paper is elaborate an LCA study of the antibacterial gel, a substance widely used during the COVID-19 pandemic, to assess the environmental impacts from its production. We focus on a case study involving the antibacterial gel from a company in Mexico. We completed the inventory analysis in collaboration with the company and compiled the impact assessments using the GaBi software and the ReCiPe method. The results shows that the principal impact categories of the antibacterial gel production are the Climate Change, Ozone Depletion, Fossil Depletion and Human Toxicity.

Keywords: Life cycle assessment · LCA · Antibacterial gel · COVID-19

1 Introduction

The Life Cycle Assessment (LCA) is a powerful tool to provide information to researchers in terms to "translate the sustainability into useful knowledge to support commercial and regulatory decision making" [1]. The begin of LCA concept start during the SETAC congress in 1990. LCA was defined as "An objective procedure for assessing the energy and environmental loads related to a process or an activity, carried out through the identification of energy and the materials used and the waste released into the environment" [2]. From this perspective, LCA was established as a methodology to evaluate the potential negative environmental impacts and the resources used all over a product life cycle (raw material extraction, design, and production process, use phases,

J. A. Marmolejo-Saucedo et al. (Eds.): COMPSE 2021, LNICST 393, pp. 12–27, 2021.
https://doi.org/10.1007/978-3-030-87495-7_2

and waste management); is a deep assessment which considers the natural ecosistems, human health, and resources [3].

The process was set up by the International Standards ISO 14040 and in specific ISO 14044. ISO 14040 and 14044 provided key principles, frameworks, and it's mandatory to develop an LCA study. The main phases which define all the steps for LCA studies are: Goal and Scope Definition, Life Cycle Inventory Analysis (LCI), Life Cycle Impact Assessment (LCIA), and Interpretation [4]. In the first phase, the main cause to perform the study, the functional unit and the limitations are included [4]. The LCI phase collect the inputs (resources) and the outputs (emissions) through the product life cycle in relation with the chosen functional unit [4]. For the LCIA phase the data from the inventory is evaluated to understand the importance of the potential environmental impacts of the studied product [4]. And to finish the LCA, in the Interpretation phase the previous values from the LCIA have a correlation with the goal and scope to reach recommendations [4].

LCA studies help to recognize the way in which products influence the environment and society, making them a real tool for companies. That is the main reason of these kinds of studies have been carried out on products of widely use such as shampoo, soaps, sunscreen, and detergents. Sanchez et al. (2018) carried out a study for the company Natura in Brazil where they make soap their product of analysis, only considering the materials for soap, packaging, and distribution [5]. Lucchetti et al. (2019) elaborated the study for the company Tea Natura in Italy analyzing the production process of a detergent, to contrast the environmental impacts with similar products [6]. Golsteijn et al. (2018) assesses the feasibility and relevance of improve Product Environmental Footprint Category Rules (PEFCR) for shampoos obviously using an LCA in European countries [7]. Thakur (2014) made a comparative study of the life cycle of sunscreen with chemical and organic products for a company in the United States [8]. The previously studies are some good examples of the great opportunity that exists within the industry and over time they will be more used to implement preventive measures and help the environment.

1.1 Alcohol-Based Hand Sanitizer

The studies of Semmelweis and Wendell established that the diseases get into the hospital were transmitted via the hands [9]. Semmelweis is considered the father of hand hygiene, and the first provider of evidence that cleansing heavily contaminated hands with an antiseptic agent can reduce the transmission of virus and germs more efficaciously than handwashing with soap and water. This statement includes the essential elements for an infection control [9].

The 80s defined a landmark in the concepts of hand hygiene in health care. The first national hand hygiene guideline was published in the starts of this years, followed by different countries over the years [10]. In 1995 the Health Infection Control Practices Advisory Committee (HICPAC) and the Center for Disease Control and Prevention (CDC) in USA, recommended the used of a waterless antiseptic agent before and after leaving the rooms of the patients [11]. In 2002, the HICPAC guidelines defined alcohol-based hand rubbing as a basic practice for hand hygiene in healthcare settings and establish that handwashing is reserved for particular situations [12].

The hand hygiene products (liquid, gel, or foam) are alcohol based. The alcohol preparation is designed for hand application to inactivate microorganisms and suppress their growth. The preparations must contain alcohol, active ingredients with excipients, and humectants [13].

The alcohol-based gel hand sanitizer varies in the amount of alcohol in its composition between 60% and 85%, the most common amount being 70% [14]. Alcohol kills between 99.99% and 99.999% of bacteria, although it does not act against spores of anaerobic bacteria, hence hydrogen peroxide is added to the gel, which it does. It is also an effective viricide and fungicide. It is characterized by the rapidity of the onset of its action (about 15 s) [14].

More recently in 2010, the Wealth Health Organization (WHO) published a Guidelines on Hand Hygiene in Health Care, this one has two sections to making alcohol-based gel hand sanitizer, a practical guide for the preparation of the formulation and the technical information. Now the people have access to important safety information, and they know the material relating to distribution [15].

Using an antibacterial hand gel has many benefits when soap and water are not available. In addition to being a simple, cheap, effective measure and within the reach of most of the population, it not only reduces the risk of infection, but also decrease the transmission of germs to other people. Nowadays, disinfection with alcohol-based products is the most quickly and effectively way to deactivating a variety of potentially harmful germs and virus in hands [15]. WHO recommends antibacterial hand gel planted the next factors [15]:

- Its microbicidal, fast and broad-spectrum activity.
- It is appropriate in remote or resource-limited locations that do not have sinks or other hand hygiene facilities (clean water, towels, etc.).
- Encourages more frequent hand hygiene, as it is faster and immediately accessible.
- Minimizes the risk of adverse effects, as it is safer, more acceptable, and better tolerated than other products.
- It reports economic benefits, since it reduces the annual cost of hand hygiene, which represents approximately 1% of the additional cost generated by infections associated with health care.

On the market there are different products that serve to eliminate bacteria and virus, for example wipes, sprays, soaps, and gels that use alcohol as an active ingredient to break the cell membrane of the microorganism or damage its structure, which tends to produce his death [16]. When purchasing antibacterial or disinfectant products, it is important to know the difference between them, the disinfectant are chemical agents used mainly on objects, in order to destroy or inhibit the growth of microbes. The antibacterial products also prevent the proliferation and development of bacteria and microorganisms harmful to health, but the term is more used in specific products for personal use [16].

The disinfectant sprays are applied with the containers in an upright position; it is sprayed on clean surfaces for 3–4 s from 15–20 cm distance. Let it rest until the surface dries. Although they are in aerosol, it is important to note that they should be used on surfaces and areas of constant contact [16]. Different from sprays or gels, disinfectant wipes are made of absorbent cellulose-based materials that are impregnated with one or more active agents. Although towels and sprays are effective, they are not recommended for the use on living tissues (such as skin), it is better to use them on surfaces such as floors, furniture, or objects because they are disinfectant products [16]. The soap should normally be applied and rubbed for a period of approximately 15 to 20 s, when washing hands, which requires the use of water to be able to use it, instead the antibacterial gel can be used immediately by putting a portion and rubbing both hands to distribute the product on the hand [16].

The antibacterial gel is the best option among the products mentioned when the hand washing is difficult, and for these advantages the demand grows little by little occupying a moderate space on pharmacy shelves. In 2020 received renewed interest due to its shortage during the COVID-19 (SARS-CoV-2) pandemic, for be one of the measures to avoid the transmission of harmful germs and virus and avoid infections [17].

1.2 COVID-19 Pandemic

COVID-19 is the disease caused by the new coronavirus known as SARS-CoV-2. The WHO know the existence of this new virus on December 31, 2019, when it was informed of a group of cases of "viral pneumonia" that had been declared in Wuhan (People's Republic of China) [18]. After it spread to all the continents of the world, it was characterized as a pandemic on March 11, 2020.

As of May 4, 2021, 153,187,889 confirmed cases (644,685 new cases) and 3,209,109 deaths (10,501 new deaths) have been reported worldwide. The overall fatality rate is 2.1% [19]. Currently America and Europe are the most affected, the first with 62,589,322 cases and the second with 52,099,114 cases [19]. This disease was registered for the first time in Mexican territory on January 14, 2020. As of May 4, 2021, 2, 352,964 total cases and 217,740 total deaths from COVID-19 have been confirmed [19].

According to the Pan American Health Organization (PAHO), informing the population about the health risks that COVID-19 may pose, as well as the measures that can be taken to protect themselves, is a key to reducing the chances that people become infected and thus mitigate further spread [20]. With the first deaths from COVID-19, the WHO disseminated health safety protocols with new hygiene and care practices that people adopted to prevent the spread of COVID-19 [20]:

- Wash your hands with soap and water.
- Use alcohol-based antibacterial gel.
- Maintain a safe distance from people.
- Use mask and face shield.
- Do not touch your face (specifically eyes, nose, and mouth).
- When you sneeze or cough, cover your mouth with a tissue or bent elbow.

This pandemic has caused an increase of more than 50% in the demand for preventive hygiene and health supplies, such as face masks, alcohol, wipes, and antibacterial gel at the beginning of the pandemic in Mexico [21]. Despite the difficulties of the health contingency, Mexico managed to position itself as an exporting country of medical products, during the first half of 2020. The exports that Mexico made to the US in 2020 are of an estimated sales value of 6 thousand 259 millions of dollars, which represented an increase of 8.4% compared to last year 2019 [22]. This represents 3.3% of exports of critical products against COVID-19 worldwide. Which establishes the country as the fifth country with the most exports of this type in the world [22].

In the list of countries that also participate in the export of products are China (54 thousand 643 million dollars), the United States (23 thousand 182 dollars), Germany (16 thousand 961 dollars) and the Netherlands (10 thousand 771 dollars). And after Mexico came Japan (5.8 billion dollars), followed by Belgium (5 thousand 596 dollars), France (5 thousand 276 dollars), Malaysia (4 thousand 440 dollars) and Ireland (4 thousand 204 of dollars) [22]. Exports from these countries represent 72.5% of global exports of medical products to face the coronavirus. Which makes them head the importance of them before the world. With the above, one has an idea of the great production that is taking place globally, and that the production, transportation, purchase, and waste will bring problems in the future if they are not conducted in the correct way [22].

1.3   Research Objective and Hypothesis

Currently, more consumers are concerned about the negative impacts that products may have, and with the help of media they have the information at their fingertips, thereby increasing a demand for products which are not harmful. The companies feel economic pressure, because people stop buying their product, and social pressure, for the change and the message they give to society.

The antibacterial gel became a product of massive use during the COVID-19 pandemic, as mentioned, according to the WHO is a crucial measure to avoid the transmission of harmful virus and avoid infections is the antibacterial gel, because is effective for destroying viruses in the hands, due to its wide capacity as a virucidal and bactericidal.

The potential environmental impacts related with its production and distribution are amplified. Later in the related work chapter it will be shown that there was no scientific information reported on the impacts that the production of the antibacterial gel generates.

The aim of this paper is elaborate an LCA study of the antibacterial gel, a substance widely used during the COVID-19 pandemic, to assess the environmental impacts from its production. It starts from the hypothesis that studying the environmental performance of antibacterial gel will allow an approximation of the environmental impact generated by its production. The limitations of the research are in accordance with the limitations of the life cycle study that will be considered in the phase one of the LCA and will be shown in the methodology chapter.

2   Related Work

The review of articles related to the LCA of the antibacterial gel production did not give the expected results, there was no scientific information reported related to this subject;

it was considered that an exhaustive review of LCA of alcohol production in general broadened the research. The production of ethyl and ethanol from another process is the most common in the papers reviewed and for research purposes they serve to know the methods and especially the environmental impacts they cause. Figure 1 shows the main articles that were considered as the state of art for this paper, this is a practical way to identify the important parts for each study, when its necessary we do not have to return to the full text and is easier to understand the LCA methodology.

Author, year	Subject and geographical context	LCA remarks and energy	Main results
Caffrey, K.R., Veal, M.W., Chinn, M.S. (2014)	Ethanol production from sweet sorghum juice in the United States.	Comparison of scenarios for a quantitative assessment of environmental issues, using the raw material for cellulosic fuel and animal feed as energy input.	A major source of cost, energy use, and environmental impacts is associated with transportation. The biomass material proposed for use in bioenergy production generally is high in moisture content and low in bulk density, reducing load capacity on a weight basis. This study showed that transportation was a major contributor to the climate change metrics, eutrophication, and solid waste landfill.
Caldeira-Pires, A., Benoist, A., Da Luz, S.M., Chaves,V., Silveira, C. M., Machado, F. (2018)	Ethanol production with sugar cane biomass in the Petrobras agro-industrial unit, in Brasilia, Brazil.	Evaluate the environmental impacts of the removal of sugarcane straw from the soil throughout the life cycle of bioethanol production, with raw material for cellulosic fuel and fossil fuel and the electrical network as energy input.	Two scenarios were studied considering the effect of the straw on the amount of sugar in the sugarcane juice and considering the use of a second-generation ethanol unit based on the hydrolysis of both bagasse and straw. In the study the main impact category was the global warming, that comes from the global climate change metrics.
Bessou, C., Lehuger, S., Gabrielle, B., Mary, B. (2013).	Ethanol production with sugar beet biomass in the Picardy region, France.	Compare ethanol from sugar beet with its fossil-based equivalent, gasoline, to examine the benefits of substituting the latter for bioethanol, albeit strictly within an attributional framework.	The sugar beet ethanol had lower impacts than gasoline for the global warming, ozone layer depletion and photochemical oxidation categories. Conversely, sugar beet ethanol had higher impacts than gasoline for acidification and eutrophication due to losses of reactive nitrogen in the arable field.
Canter, C. E., Dunn, J.B., Han, J., Wang, Z., Wang, M. (2016).	Integrated production of corn ethanol and corn stubble in the United States.	Evaluate the integrated production of ethanol from corn grains and corn stubble, using fossil fuel and the electrical network as energy input.	This analysis examines different LCA scenarios that could influence the volume of high-GHG reduction fuels that integrated corn grain-corn stover ethanol facilities produce. The main impact category in the study was global warming.
Alves, R., Guimarães, R. (2017).	Ethyl biodiesel production from soybean oil and beef tallow in a region of Brazil.	Identify the environmental impacts caused during the biodiesel production process from two different raw materials: soybean oil and bovine tallow, using fossil fuel and the electrical network as energy input.	The results show that the ethyl biodiesel production from the two different scenarios presents major environmental damage in the categories of global warming pollution, solid waste landfill, destruction of abiotic resources, destruction of the ozone layer, human toxicity, freshwater ecotoxicity, terrestrial ecotoxicity, acidification and eutrophication.

Fig. 1. Remarkable information of the papers related to the subject.

Caffrey et al. (2014) describe the ethanol production from soluble sugars recovered from sweet sorghum, implementing a comparative analysis with different process configurations. In the comparison of environmental impacts, all scenarios presented higher levels of Climate Change, Ozone Depletion and Eutrophication values for the high amount of diesel required for operations [23].

Caldeira-Pires et al. (2018) use straw together with bagasse for the production of bioethanol in two different scenarios. The evaluation is focused on the Global Warming Potential (GWP) as the main environmental impact, characterizing biotic and fossil carbon fluxes, they evaluate other impact categories such as Eutrophication and Abiotic Depletion for elements and fossil fuels [24].

Bessou et al. (2012) realize a case study involving the ethanol production from sugar beet using six different combinations of climate types and crop rotations to estimate yields and environmental emissions. Sugar beet ethanol had a lesser impact than gasoline in the Abiotic Depletion, Global Warming, Ozone Depletion, and Photochemical Oxidation categories. However, it had greater Acidification and Eutrophication impacts than gasoline. Therefore, the LCA values were sensitive to changes in management factors [25].

Canter et al. (2015) tested the difference between corn grain and stubble ethanol production considering different approaches for combined heat and power treatment. They focused on the greenhouse gas emissions (GHG) from grain ethanol. They conclude that although they have that environmental impact, there is a reduction compared to the GHG emissions from the gasoline [26].

Alves et al. (2017) compared the production of biodiesel extracted from soybean oil and bovine tallow, through the ethyl transesterification process. The data used were calculated based on similar scientific articles and nine categories of environmental impacts were analyzed for both processes, highlighting that the final evaluation shows a big damage in the categories of Destruction of Abiotic Resources, Ozone Depletion, Human Toxicity, Freshwater Ecotoxicity, Terrestrial Ecotoxicity, Acidification and Eutrophication). The biodiesel production from tallow presents a major damage in two impact categories (Land Use and Global Warming) [27].

With the previous investigation of the LCA papers related to ethanol and ethyl production, and with those mentioned within this work, the conclusion is reached that even though the studies are carried out in different places and dates, the impact categories that are the most frequently presented are Climate Change, Global Warming, Ozone Depletion, Eutrophication, and Abiotic Depletion. Based on the research, we can affirm that there is no LCA specifically focused on the antibacterial gel production.

3 Methodology

This is an LCA study of the chain production of the antibacterial gel of a Company in Mexico with national and international presence, this study follows the ISO 14044 standard. The transportation of raw material, production of the substance, pack and distribution are considered.

3.1   First Phase: Goal and Scope Definition

The goal of this study is to identify the environmental impacts caused during the production process of antibacterial gel. It starts with the transportation of raw materials from the vendor warehouse to the factory, continues with the manufacturing process of the product. After production, the antibacterial gel is packed and stored inside the factory. When the product is sold, is taken to the distribution center, when the product arrives there the study is concluded. It is considered from the perspective of the chain production of the Mexican company that we do not include the resources and emissions associated with the raw materials extraction, use, and final disposal of the product, to focus just on the environmental impacts of the antibacterial gel production is decided to skip the impact of these stages. The scope is shown in Fig. 2 that includes the process of the raw materials in the factory.

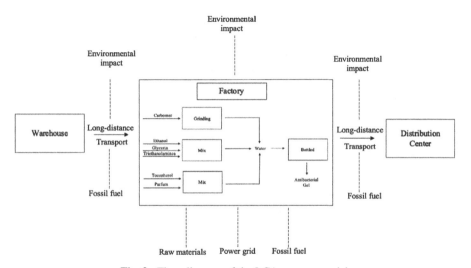

Fig. 2. Flow diagram of the LCA process model.

The reference flow is 450, 000 bottles in one day of production and the chosen functional unit is 1 bottle of 120 ml of antibacterial gel manufactured and packaged in Mexico. The company has 3 different bottle sizes for the antibacterial gel: 60 ml, 120 ml, and 450 ml. For this specific study, the 120 ml presentation was used because it is the one with the highest sales in the market.

The LCA software GaBi was used for modeling the environmental performance of the production, based on the primary data from the Mexican company along with supplementary background data from the GaBi database. GaBi is a software that models from a life cycle perspective the elements of a system to take the best decisions during the life cycle of any product [28]. GaBi combines the LCA modelling software, databases, and reporting tools [28].

The value that came from this software estimates the environmental impact categories as stated in the ReCiPe 2016 method, it was developed through a cooperation between the Dutch National Institute for Public Health and the Environment (RIVM), Radboud University Nijmegen, Norwegian University of Science and Technology, and PRé Sustainability [29]. This method is an improvement of CML 2000 and Eco-indicator 99, the principal object is transforming the life cycle inventory into indicator scores, these express the environmental impact in the corresponding impact categories [29].

3.2 Second Phase: Life Cycle Inventory Analysis (LCI)

The data given for the process managers in the factory for the inventory are identified and quantified. Antibacterial gel process data, as well as antibacterial-related information, should be meticulously collected to develop the best inventory. Is very important to have a good relationship with the concerned parties for the best data collection.

It starts defining the process stages and given them a name into the LCI, then the materials that are used in the production of the antibacterial gel, the information of each raw materials used in the process (data sheet, amount and units), the manufacturer's process, the energy consumption for each process (energy consumption pear year, origin of energy consumed and units) and the water consumption (water consumption pear year, origin of water consumed and units) must be given by the company. It must be considered if water is from storm water, treated or from the local water distribution system; the same with the energy if is from local electricity grid, solar panels, biomass, diesel. The logistic that was followed to collect the data is shows in Fig. 3, without the amount of materials for a company request. Everything collected will be used later to model the information with GaBi software to obtain life cycle impact category results.

The bottle where the substance is deposited is also part of the inventory, and the transport used to move the raw material from the vendor warehouse to the factory as well as the distances traveled, are also a vital part of the study.

When the antibacterial gel is packed and stored the final product is shipped to the distribution center.

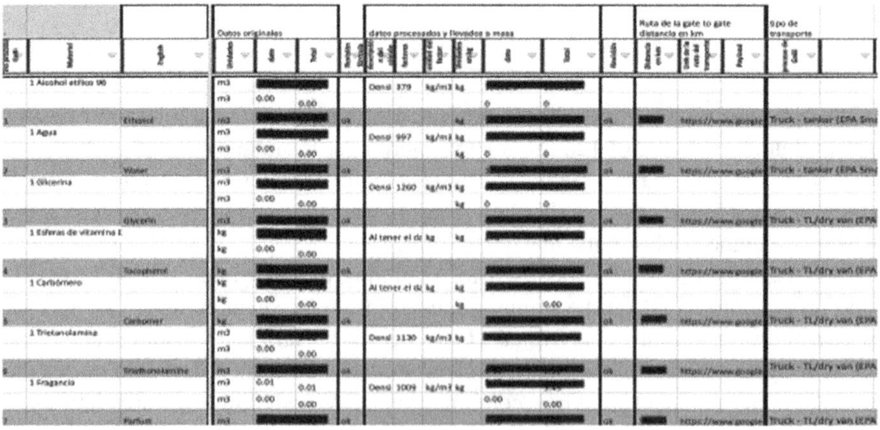

Fig. 3. The logistic of LCI used for the LCA of the antibacterial gel production.

The Fig. 4 shows the model of the process created in GaBi, the result of this will be the indicator scores express the impact categories of ReCiPe: Climate Change, Default, Excl Biogenic Carbon [kg CO2 eq.]; Climate Change, Incl Biogenic Carbon [kg CO2 eq.]; Fine Particulate Matter Formation [kg PM2.5 eq.]; Fossil Depletion [kg oil eq.]; FreshWater Consumption [m3]; Freshwater Ecotoxicity [kg 1,4 DB eq.]; Freshwater Eutrophication [kg P eq.]; Human Toxicity, Cancer [kg 1,4-DB eq.]; Human Toxicity, Non-cancer [kg 1,4-DB eq.]; Ionizing Radiation [Bq C-60 eq. to air]; Land use [Annual crop eq.·y]; Marine ecotoxicity [kg 1,4-DB eq.]; Marine Eutrophication [kg N eq.]; Metal Depletion [kg Cu eq.]; Photochemical Ozone Formation, Ecosystems [kg NOx eq.]; Photochemical Ozone Formation, Human Health [kg NOx eq.]; Stratospheric Ozone Depletion [kg CFC-11 eq.]; Terrestrial Acidification [kg SO2 eq.]; Terrestrial Ecotoxicity [kg 1,4-DB eq.] [29].

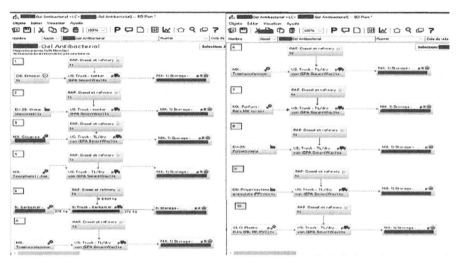

Fig. 4. Model of the antibacterial gel production in GaBi.

3.3   Third Phase: Life Cycle Impact Assessment (LCIA)

After modeling the LCI, the software rates the impacts of the second Phase in the LCA impacts categories. The data have the best approximation to the environmental impact (See Fig. 5) and the results highlight the stages that contribute the most.

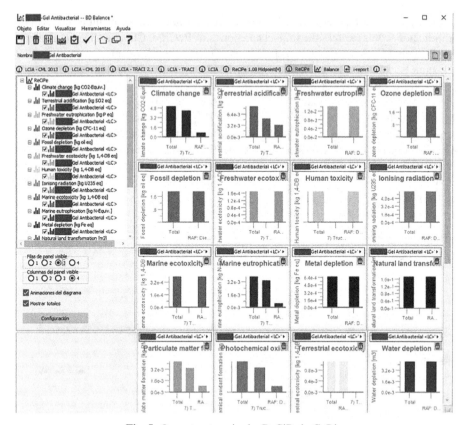

Fig. 5. Impact categories by ReCiPe in GaBi.

3.4 Fourth Phase: Interpretation

In this last phase, the impacts of the process were broken down and the interpretations obtained were verified by a critical review with the work team, this information will be developed in Sect. 4. Different improvements were proposed for the company, with the aim to reduce the environmental impacts caused by the production of its antibacterial gel. In the meeting with the process managers, they showed acceptance from the proposed changes.

4 Results and Discussion

In Fig. 6, the results of the environmental impacts in the LCA are represented in the graph.

The following table gives a better visualization of the impact categories that are consider relevant for this study, as it's prerogative in the ISO standard (Table 1).

Owing to an impact category bundle different emission into a single effect on the environment, with the program only one result can be obtained for each category, even

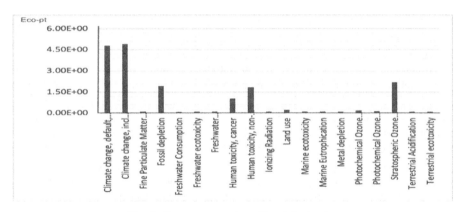

Fig. 6. Impact categories with original units.

Table 1. Impact categories.

No	Impact category		Value
1	Climate change, incl biogenic carbon	[kg CO2 eq.]	4.9E+00
2	Fine Particulate Matter Formation	[kg PM2.5 eq.]	4.26E−3
3	Fossil depletion	[kg oil eq.]	1.94E+00
4	Freshwater ecotoxicity	[kg 1,4 DB eq.]	1.69E−4
5	Freshwater Eutrophication	[kg P eq.]	1.42E−2
6	Human toxicity, cancer	[kg 1,4-DB eq.]	1.0425E +00
7	Human toxicity, non-cancer	[kg 1,4-DB eq.]	1.83E+00
8	Land use	[Annual crop eq.y]	1.7E−01
9	Marine ecotoxicity	[kg 1,4-DB eq.]	3.95E−4
10	Marine Eutrophication	[kg N eq.]	3.86E−3
11	Photochemical Ozone Formation, Ecosystems	[kg NOx eq.]	1.30E−01
12	Photochemical Ozone Formation, Human Health	[kg NOx eq.]	1.15E−01
13	Stratospheric Ozone Depletion	[kg CFC-11 eq.]	2.2E +00
14	Terrestrial Acidification	[kg SO2 eq.]	8.52E−3
15	Terrestrial ecotoxicity	[kg 1,4-DB eq.]	1.11E−3

if you have many processes. After the results, it was observed that climate change is one of the categories with the highest values in the process. This is mainly due to the data on the amount of energy consumed directly by the trucks and the machines in the chain production.

The carbon dioxide emissions emitted are caused for the transportation of the raw material from the warehouses to the factory and the final product (antibacterial gel) from the factory to the distribution centers. A fact that is worth highlighting is that although the machines are part of this negative impact, they are not the main cause of contamination, the trucks and routes of transport are the stages that polluted the most. These periodic operations and the consumption of fossil fuels are the cause of these high values.

Climate change affects the increase in radiative forcing, changing the balance of radiation and temperature control on the earth's surface, this is directly related to the depletion of the ozone layer, which would be another category that has elevated values in the study. When we have this kind of impact, it has an immediate negative effect on human health and the environment, because the emissions that are thrown into the atmosphere promote the formation of photochemical oxidants, which are gases with a powerful oxidizing effect that cause diseases and damages the ecosystem.

With the sum of the average of Climate Change, Default, Excl Biogenic Carbon and the Climate Change, Incl Biogenic Carbon, is obtained the Global Warming impact, which comes out as the main impact in the papers that were reviewed to get an idea of how the results could give to us.

As already mention, a considerable cost source and environmental impacts is associated with transportation. The category of Fossil depletion is a clear example of this, since its high values are expected due to the use of fossil fuels in freight transport, added to the fact that the distances traveled between the factory and the distribution centers can be considered relatively high in some regions. These routes contribute to the increase of particles harmful to the environment, is recommended that the routes and time in the distribution centers be optimized to improve its performance.

Although the other categories are smaller compared to the others within the same production process, they are not disposable, because even if their impact is less, it does not mean that they do not cause any damage to the environment. Each point must be considered to improve the process and lower the levels of contamination generated by the product.

The impacts of freshwater, and terrestrial ecotoxicity cause the loss of ecosystems, changing the area, bringing sudden changes in temperature, floods or, on the contrary, droughts in the area. Another impact category that has a negative contribution on the environment is eutrophication, the increase of phosphorus in the water will lead a depletion of water; even though the data does not reflect a considerable demand of water during the process and the impact category is not as representative in comparison to those already mentioned, water continues to be a vital liquid for life and must be treated with relevance.

Some actions to improve the antibacterial gel production process are the change of old truck transports and the optimization of transport routes. The implementation of new technological components that will eliminate waste and make the process more efficient are consider. In the same way, some work times were corrected in the stages within the process to improve the delivery time of the final product.

5 Conclusion

The COVID-19 pandemic caused the radical increase sales of antibacterial gel, as it became one of the measures to prevent the spread of the virus, people use it daily and several times a day. With the large amount of demand for this product, it is important to know the repercussions that its manufacture can bring to the environment. When conducting a search on this topic to inform us about the negative impacts that its production has, we realized that there were no reported results. The lack of scientific information became one of the main motivations for conducting the study.

The LCA elaborated for this work evaluated the environmental impacts of the production of antibacterial gel of a Mexican company, by documenting the experience we had with them, it is hoped that the information may be of use to other people.

The limitations for this study were that only the stages of raw material transportation, product production and transportation the final product to the distribution center were considered, to focus only on the production chain. The LCI phase was complicated, because the data collection was slow due to the confinement of the pandemic, in the same way knowing the complete production process will always be better with a visit to the factory to verify everything in depth, not only in a virtual tour like was our case.

As already mentioned, the study did not consider the part of the extraction of materials and neither was it extended to use, nor to disposal, but the importance is not ruled out. For future works it is expected to expand the work to these stages, to have the best approximation of the environmental impact of the complete life cycle of an antibacterial gel. This would be of vital importance, because the alcohol that evaporates and goes into the atmosphere must be considered, in addition to the part that goes into the water after washing hands or even knowing where the waste ends up.

We believe that conducting this kind of study is important nowadays, society's thinking is changing, more and more people are taking responsibility for their consumption, wondering which product does not pollute the environment. Finally, it is not too much to say that LCA studies have a future not only in products of widely use but also in all those that seek to improve their environmental performance.

References

1. Visentin, C., da Silva, A.W., Braun, A.B., Thome, A.: Life cycle sustainability assessment: A systematic literature review through the application perspective, indicators, and methodologies. J. Clean. Prod. **270**, 122509 (2020)
2. SETAC.: Guidelines for Life-Cycle Assessment: a code of practice. SETAC, Bruxell (1993)
3. International Standard Organization (ISO) (2006) International Standard. In: Environmental Management – Life Cycle Assessment – Principles and Framework. International Organization for Standardization. ISO 14040 (2006)
4. International Standard Organization (ISO) (2006) International Standard. In: Environmental Management – Life Cycle Assessment – Requirements and Guidelines. International Organization for Standardization. ISO 14044 (2006)
5. Ramirez, P.K.S., Petti, L., Brones, F., Ugaya, C.M.L.: Subcategory assessment method for social life cycle assessment. Part 2: application in Natura's cocoa soap. Int. J. Life Cycle Assess. **21**(1), 106–117 (2015). https://doi.org/10.1007/s11367-015-0964-x
6. Lucchetti, M.G., Paolotti, L., Rocchi, L., Boggia, A.: The role of environmental evaluation within circular economy: an application of life cycle assessment (LCA) method in the detergents sector. Environ. Clim. Technol. **23**, 238–257 (2019)
7. Golsteijn, L., et al.: developing product environmental footprint category rules (PEFCR) for shampoos: the basis for comparable life cycle assessments. Integr. Environ. Assess. Manag. **14**, 649–659 (2018)

8. Thakur, A.: Comparative Life Cycle Assessment of Sunscreen Lotion Using Organic Chemicals Versus Nano-Titanium Dioxide as UV Blocker. Arizona State University. EE.UU (2014)
9. Pittet, D.: Infection control and quality healthcare in the new millennium. Am. J. Infect. Control **33**, 258–267 (2005)
10. Simmons, B.P.: Guidelines for hospital environmental control. Section 1. Antiseptics, handwashing, and handwashing facilities. In: Centers for Disease Control and Prevention (CDC), ed. CDC Hospital Infections Program (HIP) Guidelines for Prevention and Control of Nosocomial Infections, pp. 6–10 (1981)
11. Garner, J.S.: Guideline for isolation precautions in hospitals. Infect. Control Hosp. Epidemiol. **17**, 53–80 (1996)
12. Boyce, J.M., Pittet, D.: Guidelines for hand hygiene in healthcare settings. Recommendations of the Healthcare infections Control Practices Advisory Committee and the HICPAC/APIC/IDSA Hand Hygiene Task Force. Morb. Mortal. Wkly. Rep. **51**, 1–45 (2002)
13. WHO: WHO Guidelines on Hand Hygiene in Healthcare. WHO Library Cataloguing-in-Publication Data (2009)
14. Rotter, M.: Hand washing and hand disinfection (chap. 87). In: Hospital Epidemiology and Infection Control (1999)
15. WHO: Guide to Local Production: WHO-recommended Hand rub Formulations». WHO Library Cataloguing-in-Publication Data (2010)
16. PROFECO: Analysis of disinfectant and antibacterial products. The Truth About "Germ Starters". PROFECO lab reports. Consumer magazine (2011)
17. PAHO. COVID-19: Communication material. https://www.paho.org/es/covid-19-materiales-comunicacion. Accessed 27 Feb 2021
18. WHO. Basic information about COVID-19. https://www.who.int/es/news-room/q-a-detail/coronavirus-disease-covid-19. Accessed 10 Apr 2021
19. SSA. Coronavirus COVID19 Daily Technical Release. Government of Mexico. https://www.gob.mx/salud/documentos/coronavirus-covid-19-comunicado-tecnico-diario-238449. Accessed 04 May 2021
20. PROFECO. Government of Mexico. Antibacterial Gel. An alternative at hand. https://www.gob.mx/profeco/articulos/gel-antibacterial-una-alternativa-a-la-mano?idiom=es. Accessed 29 Mar 2021
21. Forbes. Demand for facemask, alcohol, wipes, and antibacterial gel is increasing. https://www.forbes.com.mx/negocios-demanda-de-cubrebocas-alcohol-y-gel-antibacterial-sube-50-por-coronavirus/. Accessed 18 Apr 2021
22. El Economista. Mexico is the fifth supplier of medical products on US. https://www.eleconomista.com.mx/empresas/Mexico-es-el-quinto-proveedor-de-productos-medicos-para-EU-20200413-0007.html. Accessed 18 Apr 2021
23. Caffrey, K.R., Veal, M.W., Chinn, M.S.: The farm to biorefinery continuum: a techno economic and LCA analysis of ethanol production from sweet sorghum juice. Agric. Syst. **130**, 55–66 (2014)
24. Caldeira-Pires, A., Benoist, A., Da Luz, S.M., Chaves, V., Silveira, C.M., Machado, F.: Implications of removing straw from soil for bioenergy: an LCA of ethanol production using total sugarcane biomass. J. Clean. Prod. **18**, 249–259 (2018)
25. Bessou, C., Lehuger, S., Gabrielle, B., Mary, B.: Using a crop model to account for the effects of local factors on the LCA of sugar beet ethanol in Picardy region, France. Int. J. Life Cycle Assess. **18**, 24–36 (2013). https://doi.org/10.1007/s11367-012-0457-0
26. Canter, C.E., Dunn, J.B., Han, J., Wang, Z., Wang, M.: Policy implications of allocation methods in the life cycle analysis of integrated corn and corn stover ethanol production. BioEnergy Research **9**(1), 77–87 (2015). https://doi.org/10.1007/s12155-015-9664-4

27. Alves, R., Guimarães, R.: Comparing the environmental impacts of ethyl biodiesel production from soybean oil and beef tallow through LCA for brazilian conditions. Indep. J. Manag. Prod. **8**, 1285–1308 (2017)
28. SPHERA. GaBi: What is GaBi software. https://gabi.sphera.com/international/overview/what-is-gabi-software/. Accessed 28 May 2021
29. ReCiPe. ReCiPe Lyfe Cycle Assessment. https://pre-sustainability.com/articles/recipe/. Accessed 28 May 2021

An Alternative Model to Estimate Annual Budget Through TDABC Methodology in Hospitals

José Luis Hernández Arredondo[(✉)], Elí Gerardo Zorrilla Uribe, and Zaida Estafanía Alarcón Bernal

Universidad Nacional Autónoma de México, Av. Universitaria 3000, 04510 Mexico City, Mexico
josepharredondo@comunidad.unam.mx

Abstract. This work responds the Mexico City's General Hospital "Dr. Manuel Gea González" need to identify the cost behind daily operative activities. Our objective is to improve the hospital's capacity to establish a budget for its operation, to comply with the federal government's request to operate free of charge for users. To achieve the objective the authors constructed a computerized costs system, using software resources owned by the institute, based on TDABC methodology (Time Driven Activity Costing methodology), which generates and allocates expenditures depending on the execution time of a process. Likewise, the use of fuzzy logic tools helps decreasing inherent uncertainty bring by the resources consume, typical of clinical processes. It was collected information related to medical supplies, human resources, equipment, and infrastructure expenditures. This work describes the approach and execution of a pilot test made in nine clinical areas of the hospital. Finally, some proposals can guide further system development.

Keywords: TDABC · Fuzzy logic · Relational databases · Supply chain management · Healthcare system

1   Introduction

The Mexican public health care system is currently saturated due to the increasing demand for medical services, mainly because the population is getting older [1]. Therefore, there is a growth in metabolic diseases in the last years [2]. In addition, the Covid-19 pandemic saturates the system and further strains the performance of the sector at all levels. On the other hand, medical infrastructure is living an evident stagnation [3] represented by little growth for public health (in 2019 was just 2.5% of GDP) [4].

In recent years, a new policy establishes that public healthcare services must be free of charge to users [5] and a minimal private investment in comparison to other economical sectors [6] has been made.

© ICST Institute for Computer Sciences, Social Informatics and Telecommunications Engineering 2021
Published by Springer Nature Switzerland AG 2021. All Rights Reserved
J. A. Marmolejo-Saucedo et al. (Eds.): COMPSE 2021, LNICST 393, pp. 28–44, 2021.
https://doi.org/10.1007/978-3-030-87495-7_3

These factors promoted the constitution of the INSABI (Instituto Nacional de Salud para el Bienestar) in 2020, which is in charge of providing healthcare services for people without Social Security. To achieve that, the INSABI requested the hospitals update consumption data to structure expenditures of medical institutions.

The hospital "Dr. Manuel Gea González" located in Mexico City, requests a budget to the federal government authorities annually and consequently enables every process execution inside the institute. Unfortunately, it lacks an internal team dedicated to control and monitor expenses and a suitable infrastructure that allows a constant information flow from the operative areas to the strategy board. Due to the hospital's complexity, it's hard to accurately determine all the costs involved and have a model which represents with better precision the institute's behavior.

Nowadays, the Mexican Institute of Social Security (IMSS) recommends the use of a costing model based on two approaches: first takes information in an up-to-down method and allocate total costs into productive areas (in this case, clinical departments) proportional to the volume of production, that means areas with more work, will have assigned more budget. The second part obtains detailed information from each operational department, guided by an Activity Based Costing (ABC), where every process mapped and then consumed resources allocated according to the specific needs of each one. In aggregation, we can obtain a more accurate model compared to using only one approach at a time. This methodology was established and explained in 2011 [7] in an attempt to standardize the way hospital calculate their annual budget.

The studied hospital belongs to the IMSS infrastructure, so it was crucial to implement the costing guide provided by the Institute. However, this approach has a high human and time resource consumption because usually, the staff has to dedicate a substantial amount of time to analyze and register the processes' performance. For that reason, in 2004, the Health Ministry designed and distributed a computational tool to help the cost estimation of hospitals based on Microsoft Excel [8]. Unfortunately, the program code is obsolete to modern software platforms and hard to reimplement to the hospital.

Usually, the healthcare institutions that do not belong to the IMSS infrastructure, have a different costing structure that is not standardized. This consists of an approach of the annual budget requisitions with a hybrid of the method applied in the IMSS and a Traditional Costing System, which implies the direct allocation of expenses to the given services and calculates the number of cases they had in a year and sum the overhead costs. This kind of structure implies a big accuracy error in the estimated budget.

Those are one of the main reasons the authors proposed a new structure, adapted to the hospital circumstances, to obtain data more easily from clinical areas, reduce the time that information is processed, and mainly, have more precision about the total expenses generated by the hospital, only using software resources owned by the institute because of the project's limited budget. The result was the development of three elements: first of all, the use of a methodology established by R. Kaplan in 2004 named Time-Driven Activity-Based Costing (TDABC)[9][1] which is characterized by determining expenses depending on the execution time of activities, where each one has a cost rate per unit of time; moreover, it was necessary to design and construct a database with formularies that allowed the capture of consumption data for all clinical areas; and third, all this conducted by an established plan from project management theory.

In this document, we explain some details of the mentioned system, from the theoretical approach to the computer program in charge of database management. In the next section, we will explain the TDABC theory and how it works in a variant oriented to the healthcare industry. In the same way, we will talk about the fuzzy inference used to diminish uncertainty, both on medical supplies consumption quantity and execution time for all the different processes. Later in the same section will be an application on "Dr. Manuel Gea González" hospital, where it talks about the method adaptations made due to the institutional context. In the Results section, we will discuss obtained values from the nine studied areas and particularities that emerged in each case, in addition to some data related to departments' efficiency. Finally, in the Conclusions section, we will describe implementation challenges the team faced, and therefore possible improvements in favor of system performance.

1.1   Previous Work

After Kaplan and Anderson created the TDABC method in 2004 [9] various authors put it into practice because of its implementation simplicity. TDABC is an evolution of the original ABC (Activity Based Costing) method [10] oriented to the manufacturing industry, but it turns hard to apply when the processes are not standardized (we can see a deep comparative between methods on del Rio [11]). Demeere uses TDABC, which in 2009 [12] apply the methodology to a clinic in Belgium (to five different departments), the study highlights the great adaptability, as well as the vision granted to the hospital's strategic level. After, in 2011 Kaplan [13] launch a variant of the method made specially to hospitals, centered on following patient's "cycle of care", where integrates all the processes used by patients in a specific medical condition. This method was applied at the University of Texas MD Anderson Cancer Center in 2010 by H. Albright [13, pp. 61–64], where we can find the importance of physicians' awareness about the cost born from treating patients.

Dr. Öker [14] points the need to increase productivity in the healthcare sector. For that reason, she concludes the TDABC method as an alternative to face a fast-changing reality and a tool with great precision obtained from allocating costs in just one variable, time. McLaughlin [15] sees an opportunity to redesign processes in mutual agreement because everyone sits on the same table analyzing better ways to improve the system. Bakhtiar Ostadi proposed on 2019 [16] an approach to TDABC, where use tools from Fuzzy inference to obtain resources cost, time, and capacity values. The goal is to reduce uncertainty and

---

[1] an evolution of ABC costing.

have more reliable information. On the other hand, A. Martin [17] emphasizes the challenges of implementing it because it is imperative to have an updated resource platform also, the natural resistance from healthcare providers being transparent in reporting their daily tasks. Finally, G. Keel & et al. [18] revised 25 TDABC applications, as same as Ganesh [19], independently they conclude the difficulties determining indirect costs (there is no way of proceeding on Kaplan original method). Nevertheless, they can identify some benefits like operational improvements, reduction of resource waste, and lead time decrease. An approach to defining a starting work structure is the Guide to Public Health Supply Chain Costing [20], where we can find some steps to consider when someone estimates costs on health care institutions.

2   Method

2.1   Technological Tools

The constricted resources and budget of the hospital let available just a few resources for innovation, especially the technological infrastructure. Nevertheless, there was the availability of a Microsoft license and the feasibility of a friendly user interface. The project required to be enhanced using technological tools, that would improve the method to be organized and automatized, so it can make the data link without the common employee error interaction. With that in mind, it was analyzed the use of Microsoft Access as the most reliable solution to attend all the demands. As well as it has the most advantages: solid database software structure, availability of the license in all the computers, feasibility to be managed through a central server connected to all the devices in the hospital, and the easiness of customer usage.

The lack of knowledge and experience in developing technological tools that could improve the process realization was a major constraint in the hospital employee and administrative capabilities. Administrative departments could facilitate the few available resources, but there was not much time they could invest. Therefore, the authors developed a project plan to build an Access database that stores and computes the core information. We expected two different users: medical employees (who would feed the database) and control users (who would manage stored data). Hence, the construction of Access forms through Visual Basic code was critical. So that users were able not only to give data but also interact with the available information. In addition, the database is attached to an Excel sheet, built to combine the core information inside the Access database about processes and resources consumption relationships. Hence, it can be computed more efficiently than inside Access and would display the results of the method showing strategic financial information and becomes more user-friendly with the chief executives of the institution for its interpretation and usage.

In resume, the method was enhanced by the usage of:

Access database obtains, manages, and controls the information about resources' consumption in the hospital. Excel form analyzes, computes the

Access' database information. In consideration of the designed costing method and displays strategic information about the hospital financial requirements.

2.2   Application

The hospital used to work with two flow stream budget revenue, one from cost per service charged to the patients, and the other was an annual budget allocated by the federal government. The new public healthcare policies detonate a need to restructure the service to achieve universal free cost healthcare services. Therefore, the government set new tasks to capture and analyze the expenses of each institution that give attention to people without social insurance.

Nevertheless, the growing and aging population of Mexico represents a latent problem. In addition to the increase of non-transmissible metabolic diseases, such as diabetes and hypertension. That requires high levels of investment and enhances the capability of the public healthcare services throughout the years. Those demands will stretch the current system and the need for a new methodology to know how much expenses allocate in each type of disease [21].

The risk involved in a wrong executed budget could put at risk all the hospital's operability. Hence, they know that with the new government policy, they shall adequate their assigned budget. Nevertheless, they had no infrastructure and human capabilities to develop an advanced costing system, only the traditional time sequence forecasting method, which has proven wrong several times. Hence, the authors developed an adaptation from the TDABC methodology according to the hospital's resources and capabilities. In addition, it was applied project management theory to define and plan task sequences, goals, and objectives expected from this project. As well as quality, stakeholders, and a work breakdown structure that allowed control and project performance follow and their stakeholders, decreasing the level of project execution uncertainty.

In the case study, the authors and the hospital chief executives decided to apply the method in a pilot group considering nine clinical departments: Anesthesiology, Blood bank, Stomatology, Internal Medicine, Neonatology, Nutrition, Ophthalmology, Rehabilitation, and Urology. In addition, of support and administrative departments of the hospital that influences the resource consumption interaction of the clinical department. The four analyzed resources for the costing system were: infrastructure, human resources, equipment, and medical supplies. The new method based on the TDABC technique consists of the following steps:

- Mapping Activities
- Resources Group identification
- Departments total cost
  - Contracts assignment
  - Human resources assignment
  - Infrastructure assignment
  - Equipment classification and assignment
  - Cost assignment
- Department's workforce capacity

- Capacity rate
- Processes execution time
- Cost per activity

Mapping activities is the first step in the TDABC technique used in this article. It was analyzed all the activities that the different departments execute. Those processes were reviewed, analyzed, and modified to obtain the most representative processes of the patient care chain of each department, considering the type of capabilities that each service offers to the patients. The processes were reviewed considering the following question parameters

- The process is still functional?
- The frequency of process realization is still representative?
- Is still the best available process for the cycle care of the patient? Is it antique or old?
- The process is too general, it encloses too many procedures or processes that will be better as separate processes
- The process is very similar to a different one, causing redundancies
- It is possible to fusion similar processes as one, because the activities are very similar or are part of the same clinal procedure
- The process has very diverse outcomes hanging on the type of patients, it will be representative to classify this process in consideration of the type of outcome.

This mapping process was managed by a healthcare professional of each department in which the method will be applied.

In the Resource Group (RG) identification the aim is to enclose all similar costs that can exist between services. A resource consumption classification was made in consideration of the hospital functional structure, type of processes, and clinical departments. Hence, the criteria used for this step was to classify all the processes in consideration of their department and the amount of time and resources consumption. This step analysis shall be made with the collaboration of healthcare professionals, healthcare executives of the hospital, and the implementation team. As a result, it was established 5 RG: Surgical, Outpatient, Diagnostic, Ambulatory Surgery, Therapeutic.

In terms of standardized procedures, the authors suggest establishing for each of these RG a description, so it becomes easier the next processes classification step. After the RG elaboration, all the processes of the 9 clinical departments were classified according to the established Resource Groups, which depends on the clinical nature of each process. This classification is called "divisions", so it becomes easier to distinguish the consumption of available resources in a general way, that can differentiate between big cost differences.

Until here, it was structured the elements that will work as the drivers to have general components with the right level of specificity in the amount of resource consumption, with the cost as the main parameter of segregation. Therefore, the method is specific enough in the big difference, but as general as it can be to make it easier and cheaper the implementation. The resources assignment in each department is key to the good implementation of the method. It is required good communication and collaboration between the administrative departments to have access to all the financial and resource information. As it was required information in terms of contracts, employees, procurement, equipment, inventory, infrastructure, and medical supplies.

Through the Plan and Integration Department of the general hospital, we obtain all the required information of:

- Human resources
    - Assigned Area
    - Salary
    - Schedule and Laboral days
    - Type of professional
- Inventory
    - Clinical mobiliary
    - Medical equipment
    - Office equipment
    - Nonclinical mobiliary
    - Vehicles
- Infrastructure
    - Building plans
    - Assigned area to each department
- Contracts
    - Maintenance
    - Procurement
    - Outsourcing
    - Insurance
- Medical Supplies o Prices per product and per minimum quantity.

The human resources were classified according to the type of professional and salary differences. The salary of the existent types of employees in the hospital was reviewed. Therefore, since it existed not a significant difference in the amount, the professionals were assigned according to the hospital information, where it was specified the quantity of each professional that each department has. So, the data was upload to the database, then the logic of it, classified and assigned the type of professional, the quantity and the salary per year and per employee of all the professionals of each department.

For the inventory was designed a classification system in terms of the type of equipment, classified by the description, usage, and complexity of technology. It was established 5 types of equipment:

- Life support equipment
- Surgical equipment
- Therapeutic equipment
- Diagnostic and monitoring equipment
    - Low technological complexity

- Medium technological complexity
- High technological complexity
- Others
  - Clinical mobiliary
  - Nonclinical mobiliary

The hospital inventory describes all the material assets, where are placed, and when they were acquired. The depreciation value allocates as the only way to assign a cost of the equipment. Nevertheless, because of the public healthcare constraints, most of the hospital equipment is quite old, causing that it was required to modify the standard depreciation values Thus, it was established to consider all the equipment with less than 20 years of being acquired, and the following depreciation values: 10% for others and therapeutic, 12.5% for surgical and low and medium technological complexity diagnostic and monitoring equipment, 20% for life support and high technological complexity.

The parameters were uploaded into the Access database and the system classifies the data given according to all the requirements established and extracts the depreciation value and assigned the cost to their corresponding department.

Meanwhile, the contract information was segregated and assigned, according to the contract description and type of service, through an Access form in a manual way. Since it exists different procurement, outsourcing and service provider the assignation was supervised by personal with hospital's administrative knowledge. The main criteria were that the cost of the contract was attributed to the corresponding department that manages, deploys, or consumes this type of resource/service. This amount shall correspond to an annual operating cost sum, the database makes the relation of the specific contract and the department assigned.

The difference in terms of hospital infrastructure costs is quite significant since we have common areas that are used not only for administrative and support departments but also in outpatient processes. In contrast, the infrastructure used for specialized clinical processes such as surgical, diagnostic, and hospitalization procedures is more expensive than the common areas. As a result, two types of infrastructure: general and clinical areas should exist.

In this concept was attributed the cost that corresponds to the depreciation of the infrastructure, maintenance employees and contracts, insurance, electrical and water fees, so on and so forth. Those concepts build the general fee of the infrastructure that was divided by the total amount of square meters of the hospital. The process was automatically achieved through the database and obtains an amount of money per square meter.

The cost of medical gas contracts, clinical infrastructure depreciation, and clinical contracts was summed by the database and divided by the total square meters of clinical areas of the hospital. Operating rooms, hospitalization areas, and diagnostic/laboratory areas build the clinical areas. Then, was obtained a medical per square meter fee. The general square meter fee acts as the base for the clinical fee since it makes use of all the common infrastructure of the hospital.

The clinical per square meter fee was the result of the sum of the general fee and the medical per square meter fee.

The information of the medical supplies was realized in a previous stage of the work and was only extracted uploaded to the database. This information corresponds to a fuzzy logic procedure for estimating the medical supplies consumption of all the processes of the clinical department. The medical supplies correspond to medicament, reactive, materials and all the medical resources that are used in a disposal way to provide the clinical service.

All the cost of human resources, equipment, and infrastructure was automated summed by the database to each one of the corresponding administrative and clinical departments that were considered in the pilot group. The cost of each one of those elements attends to a one-year usage period. In other words, one year of salary, one year of depreciation, one year of medical supplies usage (according to the number of procedures that were notified in a year of biostatistics), one year of infrastructure usage. The data was uploaded and warehoused in the database for future disposal. In the next step, we will start talking about the main denominator and control element of the method.

As told, it has been built and enclosed most of the characteristics and elements that have a direct cost associated with providing healthcare services to each of the administrative and clinical departments. Nevertheless, it is critical in the original TDABC to have a time control element that provides the cost segregation detail needed, in terms of the real utilization of all those resources. The cost rates assume this role, they are based on the time utilization of each process. But first, it is needed to know the cost rate of each department, and here is where the great differentiation point of each department is built since we make it throughout the available workforce time of each department.

At this point we need to define the criteria used for considering or not the workforce, for this case of study it was stated the following criteria for considering it as part of the available workforce time: All the healthcare professionals that work directly with the patient. In other words, all the professionals that their interaction adds value to the patient in the care chain, e.g. physicians, nurses, auxiliary clinicians, so on so forth. Those with administrative or support roles were not considered for the workforce availability of the clinical departments, but all the employees were considered in the administrative department's workforce time.

Differentiate the workforce in Theoretical time which is the sum of all the Laboral hours of the selected professionals time, and a real-time that employs the theoretical time but with a factor of discount that represents the idle time of the employees such as mealtime, bathroom, and other activities that are not related with the patient but are made during the work time.

The database information about the human resources includes the data about the days they work and the time they need to work it was easier in the database to make the sum about the available workforce time per department in consideration of the described criteria. Nevertheless, in the hospital, there are 3 types of contracts: interns, base, and confidence, and four turns: morning, evening, night, and special. Each one of these with different employee benefits in terms of non-working days and holiday periods. So, through an Excel algorithm that analyzes the type of contract from the employees established all the Laboral days that they should work. With the information of the Laboral days per year and Laboral time per day per professional was established the theoretically available workforce time per year and per employee. Then, all the employee's time information of each department was summed in the database and was given the theoretical workforce time per year and per department. Secondly, must be applied the discount of idle time, in this case, was established that the real workforce time is 80% of the theoretical time, so this value was applied through the database to obtain the real workforce time in hours per year and per department.

At this point, the database has collected all the information about the operational direct cost and available workforce time of each department per year. Therefore, the first calculation of the method was obtained: the capacity rate. The capacity rate is defined as the cost per unit of time of executing any activity in the department. It is obtained through the division of the sum of all the operational direct costs of the described resources per year divided by the total real available workforce hours of the same department. This is the moment in which the database links the information to an Excel spreadsheet that was designed to extract and make de division and obtain the capacity rate of each department per hour since it was the case main time unit driver. The spreadsheet obtains automatically all the information and calculates it for all the departments.

The process execution time is one of the core activities and most demanding processes of the method. Acts as a core element to the required execution time of all the processes of the clinical departments. The Access forms worked as the interactive interface where the healthcare professional of each department was assigned to introduce and feed with their time data the system. The time needed for each process of their respective department. To avoid uncertainty, it was applied a fuzzy inference method with the usage of a triangular function. Therefore, it was demanded that they provide 3 values of the time employed: an optimistic time when the patient responds well and the process is quite easy, the meantime in their experience, and the fatalistic time when the patient complicates and does not respond well to the process and requires the most time of it. The mathematical method was expressed on the Excel spreadsheet and obtain the data from the Access forms that compute all the information to obtain the fuzzy inference value of time of each process. In addition to the process's time, it was also used the fuzzy inference on the medical supply resource consumption to avoid the uncertainty of the specific amount of those supplies used in each process. The fuzzy inference makes use of the Yager index through the expected value to give an approximation of the behavior of the expected number.

The assignation of the cost of each process represents the final step. Escalate it to the operational cost per department is critical to obtain a budget estimate. Hence, it was designed the logic of it. As it is known the operative processes work as a combination of direct and indirect activities. Those indirect can be defined as support processes, e.g. biomedical assistance, or a surgical or ambulatory department intervention on the process execution. To make representative those support areas process in the interaction with the main clinical processes it was assigned to a hospital administrative and clinical professional to fill an interaction table where it was defined all the supportive areas that were found in the hospital. Then, the professional had to link for each process which of those areas were related in the process and an estimated percentage. As a result, is built the relational table that represents the usage of the support department of all the processes from the pilot clinical departments.

Once more is applied the Resource Group definition, at this point in the method we have a general fee of cost per unit time of each department. Until now is explained how was made the cost segregation of each resource group in terms of the equipment used for each process. In other words, as an example, if we are talking about a surgical process it will correspond to a surgical RG. So, its fee will be based on the general cost of the department plus all the equipment and infrastructure required for a surgical process (clinical area and surgical equipment in this example) and a new total cost of the surgical RG of this specific department is obtained (based on the general operating cost) that is different from the resource used for a therapeutic process. This is a Resource Group cost segregation it's made automatically in the cost rate step but is explained now to be more representative about how the costing process is differentiated. Hence, even when the method looks too general it was designed to make the representative differentiation in key steps.

With that in mind now we have cost fees per hour per each department's Resource Group. So now in the excel spreadsheet, the cost is built. For every process of the clinical departments make the following procedure:

- Extract the type of RG of the process
- It extracts the rate of the specific department Resource Group
- Analyze the relational table and extracts the name of the support departments that are related to the process
- Extract the rate per hour of those related departments
- Sum the rate per hour of the specific department Resource Group of the process and the rate per hour of the related support departments and is obtained a process rate value
- Obtain the information of the fuzzy inference time value obtained for that specific process in hours
- Multiple the process rate value and the fuzzy inference time value to obtain an expected cost per process realized
- Is extracted the amount of money required in medical supplies for this process and is summed to the cost per process and is obtained a total cost per process
- Information from biostatistics about the quantity of realized processes per year of this type is extracted
- The information about the quantity of made processes per year is multiplied by the total cost per process and is obtained an estimated operating process cost per year.

This procedure is realized for every process in the clinical departments and then it is summed all the estimated operating process costs per year of all the processes of each department to obtain an estimated annual operating cost of the department. Finally, we summed all the clinical departments' annual operating costs to the cost of the administrative departments (e.g. directions, financial, legal, etc.), and an estimated budget can be estimated for the hospital.

3   Results

Taking into consideration the resources from contracts and ledgers before mentioned, we distributed expenses into two groups; direct costs, which include all the processes around the nine studied clinical areas, these activities treat patients directly in one or another way; on the other hand, we have indirect costs, which include all administrative work and activities not making patient's direct care attention. In the first group, the model calculates a need of MXN 315,231,406.45 (USD 16,369,364.83)[2] to provide the services from the nine areas for one year; for indirect costs, it takes MXN 203,658,187.54 (USD 10,575,580.68)for operate normally along one year; in total the hospital expenses are MXN 518,889,593.99 (USD 26,944,945.52)[3].

For more detail we will show particular quantities for each clinical area:

Table 1. Costs and efficiencies related to each clinical area

Department	Annual cost (MXN)	Efficiency (%)	Cost rate
Anaesthesiology	$83,277,829.87	101.99	401.31
Blood bank	$48,957,638.95	206.63	455.78
Stomatology	$51,949,286.39	252.85	483.74
Internal medicine	$ –	–	683.57
Neonatology	$54,121,884.38	44.75	1855.90
Nutrition	$37,652,114.93	292.85	266.83
Ophthalmology	$17,684,786.10	23.18	445.10
Rehabilitation	$8,267,668.78	87.41	309.90
Urology	$13,320,197.04	56.66	893.27

The second column costs of the Table 1 come from the sum of all processes performed in one year, 2019 in this case, so main expenses are on Anaesthesiology area being of MXN 83,277,829.87 (USD 4,324,458.64), the minimum was

---

[2] Using the annual 2019 average dollar exchange rate of 1 USD = 19.2574 MXN, year of analyzed hospital's data.

[3] It's important to say that this number does not represent all expenditures the hospital have along one year, because we are just taking into consideration costs from the nine clinical areas studied in this pilot test.

Rehabilitation with MXN 8,267,668.78 (USD 429,324.24). Also, the third column represents the calculated departments' efficiency, i.e., the quotient between the available theoretical workforce and the actual work done by the areas (we have to remember this variable is obtained directly from the time expended on processes of each department), all of this represented in time units. In cases where the efficiency is higher than 100% means that the area is executing work that exceeds their capacity in terms of workforce or machines, the strategic board has to implement actions to improve their work, that is the case for Stomatology with 252.85% or Nutrition with 292.85%. On the other hand, we have percentages less than 100% in this case the area have more staff than they need for their daily activities, in this case, we have to look out Ophthalmology having 23.18% or Urology at 56.66%. The adequate interpretation of the efficiency results needs are dependent of the accuracy of the needed time for process execution. Finally, in the last column, we can appreciate the rate cost per time unit, which shows how much cost change depending on the medical supplies, staff, and equipment usage between departments. This information provides an outlook of where it is draining the hospital income.

Table 2. Annual cost of processes

Process	U. cost (MXN)	Annual frequency	Annual cost (MXN)
General Anaesthesia	1,567.75	7968	43,721,471.83
Serologic test	1,818.67	4794	31,677,944.85
Orthodontic treatment	2,063.49	7125	29,894,754.65
Sedation	6,476.24	1200	20,205857.09
Enteral nutrition	2,447.26	3284	19,442,270.90
Parenteral nutrition	2,033.21	2660	13,070,181.98
Membrane rupture treatment (infection)	26,837.49	50	12,881,993.26
Intrathecal block	1,429.98	3093	12,826,472.84

Starting from the Table 2 above, we can observe some of the most expensive processes annually, highlights "General Anaesthesia" presumably due to their supplies cost. Remember, the annual cost of procedures is defined by multiplying the rate from the area and the frequency the task is executed along the year (also, the sum of supplies cost utilized is counted). It appears to be some consistency in costs around 11 million MXN annually, except for the upper elements which, consume a considerable part of the operational budget (19–43 million MXN annually). In some cases, the annual cost rises because of the high number of process repetitions during the year; in other cases, the elevated cost of a unitary process translates into a substantial annual cost.

As we can see, this method saves expended resources on implementation because the algorithm distributes and estimates consumption from each area depending on declared information in accounting books. We achieve this by combining data from statistical and accounting departments with detailed supply consumption data directly from the clinical workforce. Instead of mapping every activity (like the ABC method) and attach their resource use, the method manages all expenses in "Resource Groups", which have a rate cost per use time. If we have the execution time from each activity, we can obtain the total cost from processes and departments. Also, the computational tool is in charge of doing the calculations, allowing physicians to concentrate on minimal administrative activities but delivering accurate and updated data for better decision making.

In addition, the use of fuzzy logic tools improves the system performance, especially for the healthcare environment, because usually, it is hard to define standards on medical practice due to inherent uncertainty. Compared to traditional ABC or Monte Carlo simulation, these tools behave more efficiently and reflect activities under uncertain conditions adequately, that is because this approach is easier to understand for physicians when is expressed in terms of critical, common, and optimistic scenarios. All of this fits perfectly with the public healthcare sector circumstances where the demand is increasing at a high rate, the diseases are becoming more expensive and the institutions' performance is more challenging due to clinical and management problems. Therefore, this kind of work will help all the public healthcare institutions where the budget is constrained and does not have the flexibility to invest time and money in developing new operating strategies.

3.1 Discussion

There is no Internal Medicine information in the Table 1 because no data was delivered to us about the annual quantity of processes by the department when we write the official report. Moreover, we saw some inconsistency in the data previously acquired, being necessary to redefine resources consumed and establish a new mapping in the area; something impossible at that moment because Mexico was on his worst stage of the COVID-19 pandemic, and all activities from Internal Medicine were interrupted and focused attending the patients.

The equipment depreciation method also was modified compared to the traditional method used in the hospital, there is a lot of equipment that should have been replaced long time ago, nevertheless, the constraints in resources forces to the institution to make use of this equipment and increase expected service life time of it. The depreciation was adapted to the accountability reality of the institution, so there was equipment that could make a cost difference between the processes.

When we presented the results to hospital authorities, they disagreed about the Neonatology efficiency results because there is one of the busiest specialties in the hospital. So, after reviewing the information provided from the area, we concluded there are other processes or activities they do but don't report because it is an emergency area and results in complicated perform bureaucratic tasks due to the nature of their work.

On the other hand, we had problems with supplies but mainly with General Anaesthesia. Because we use a hospital register that they already have for all the medical supplies commonly use, so in many cases, there was no relation between the quantities they use and its units (in other words, the supply units, like milliliters or grams, didn't match consistently with the quantities areas report they use). That causes a divergence of information and prices out of reality, so we have to eliminate those atypical elements meanwhile the hospital polish their registers.

4   Conclusions

Through this work were identified some Mexican healthcare system needs. So, a first step to transform the actual circumstances is to be clear on the amount of money the institutions will need to operate normally and detect opportunity areas more efficiently. In addition, our solution approach raises awareness of physicians in how the resources are consumed, provoking a better use and attempts to optimize their consumption. To tactical groups emerge ideas of restructuring their processes for delivering a better service, generated when the entire context spectrum is showed. Finally, we can highlight the benefits of cost estimate systematization since it gives a preamble to standardize activities and makes internal transactions more transparent also, this is a tool to the strategic sphere with which they can make better long-term decisions.

The system constructed was made to self-manage if the hospital decides to implement it to the rest departments and intended to be as easy as possible for principal users, physicians who are non-experts on software development. At first, we noticed natural resistance in adopting this new approach from the hospital's staff. But through the project, people were increasingly interested in final results, provoking a better response from clinical areas and obtaining reliable data due to their cooperation. For that reason, we think these are the initial steps of an evolving system that could be functional not just for Gea González Hospital but the entire network of 2nd and 3rd level healthcare institutions that grants a smooth and constant information flow in favor of our final users who deserve an incessant search of new ways to offer a better service, the patients of the Mexican healthcare system.

4.1   Future Work

As we mentioned, this is a preamble in search of strengthening and refining the interface constructed. In that way, some proposals could be interesting to implement in new future projects. At first, database and system logic were established on the Microsoft environment, manly Excel and Access, but during the project, the hospital was managing the purchase of MySQL licenses, so it is advisable to export all data to that platform, even more, if they are planning to scale the system to all the hospital. Likewise, we don't have to forget to make a periodical revision about the resource validity because they change constantly. For that reason, it's necessary to automate or improve the way the system process these transactions. On the other hand, we recommend a deeper analysis for processes and their relations between clinical areas, because in that way we can define clearly the critical patient paths of their attention cycle and optimize resources allocation. A dedicated team to this system could enhance it by giving it maintenance and improving the process mapping in terms of resource and time consumed in each process. At the end, this should be a task that needs to detonate a new accountability and control culture in which every stakeholder in the hospital should align their data management to this system so it can be enhanced to its maximum potential. Finally, this is an always-changing ecosystem, so the computerized costs program has to update its data until reaching a higher degree of convergence with actual hospital behavior and obtain trustworthy information that allows an excellent sustainable performance.

Acknowledgements. We thank to CIMA (Applied Medical Innovation Center) department at General Hospital "Dr. Manuel Gea González", specially to Edna Rangel who greatly supported the development of this project and to Miguel Gorostieta who helped us obtaining the hospital information from managers and directors. Also, we thank UNAM (Autonomous Mexico's National University) and its PAPIIT program IA105220 "Optimización en Logística Hospitalaria" for support and make possible the project.

References

1. López, M.F.H.: La situación demográfica en México. Panorama desde las proyecciones de población, p. 10 (2013)
2. Ávila Burgos, L., Serván-Mori, E., Wirtz, V.J., Sosa-Rubí, S.G., Salinas-Rodríguez, A.: Efectos del Seguro Popular sobre el gasto en salud en hogares mexicanos a diez años de su implementación. Salud Pública México **55**(Supl. 2), 91 (2013). http://saludpublica.mx/index.php/spm/article/view/5103
3. Sosa-Rubí, S.G., Sesma, S.: ANí lisis del gasto en salud en México, p. 42
4. Velázquez, M.: Presupuesto Público para Salud 2020, October 2019. https://codigof.mx/presupuesto-publico-para-salud-2020/
5. de Salud, S.: ACUERDO de Coordinación para garantizar la prestación gratuita de servicios de salud, medicamentos y demás insumos asociados para las personas sin seguridad social en los términos previstos en el Título Tercero Bis de la Ley General de Salud, que celebran la Secretaría de Salud, el Instituto de Salud para el Bienestar y la Ciudad de México (2020)
6. Gobierno de Mexico: Acuerdo nacional de inversión en infraestructura del sector privado, November 2019
7. Subsecretaría de Integración y Desarrollo del Sector Salud: Manual institucional y guía sectorial para la aplicación de la mtedología de costos, September 2011

8. Dirección General de Planeación y Desarrollo en Salud: Módulo de estimación de costos hospitalarios (2004)

9. Kaplan, R.S., Anderson, S.R.: Time-Driven Activity-based Costing: A Simpler and More Powerful Path to Higher Profits, p. 220

10. Cooper, R., Kaplan, R.S.: Activity-based systems: measuring the costs of resource usage. Acc. Horizons **6**, 1–13 (1992)

11. del Rio Blanco, N.: Comparison between ABC and TDABC. Actual practical application. Leon, Spain, July 2015

12. Demeere, N., Stouthuysen, K., Roodhooft, F.: Time-driven activity-based costing in an outpatient clinic environment: development, relevance and managerial impact. Health Policy **92**(2–3), 296–304 (2009). https://linkinghub.elsevier.com/retrieve/pii/S0168851009001316

13. Kaplan, R.S., Porter, M.E.: How to solve the cost crisis in health care. Harv. Bus. Rev. **89**(9), 47–64 (2011)

14. Öker, F., Özyapici, H.: A new costing model in hospital management: time-driven activity-based costing system. Health Care Manager **32**(1), 23–36 (2013). https://journals.lww.com/00126450-201301000-00004

15. McLaughlin, N., et al.: Time-driven activity-based costing: a driver for provider engagement in costing activities and redesign initiatives. Neurosurg. Focus **37**(5), E3 (2014). https://thejns.org/view/journals/neurosurg-focus/37/5/article-pE3.xml

16. Ostadi, B., Mokhtarian Daloie, R., Sepehri, M.M.: A combined modelling of fuzzy logic and Time-Driven Activity-based Costing (TDABC) for hospital services costing under uncertainty. J. Biomed. Inform. **89**, 11–28 (2019). https://linkinghub.elsevier.com/retrieve/pii/S153204641830220X

17. Martin, J.A., Mayhew, C.R., Morris, A.J., Bader, A.M., Tsai, M.H., Urman, R.D.: Using time-driven activity-based costing as a key component of the value platform: a pilot analysis of colonoscopy, aortic valve replacement and carpal tunnel release procedures. J. Clin. Medi. Res. **10**(4), 314–320 (2018). http://www.jocmr.org/index.php/JOCMR/article/view/3350

18. Keel, G., et al.: Time-driven activity-based costing for patients with multiple chronic conditions: a mixed-method study to cost care in a multidisciplinary and integrated care delivery centre at a university-affiliated tertiary teaching hospital in Stockholm, Sweden. BMJ Open **10**(6), e032573 (2020). https://bmjopen.bmj.com/lookup/doi/10.1136/bmjopen-2019-032573

19. Ganesh, L.: Impact of indirect cost on access to healthcare utilization. Int. J. Med. Sci. Public Health **4**(9), 1255 (2015). http://www.scopemed.org/fulltextpdf.php?mno=178179

20. McCord, J., Tien, M., Sarley, D.: Guide to public health supply chain costing: a basic methodology (2013)

21. Tremmel, M., Gerdtham, U.-G., Nilsson, P., Saha, S.: Economic burden of obesity: a systematic literature review. Int. J. Environ. Res. Public Health **14**(4), 435 (2017). http://www.mdpi.com/1660-4601/14/4/435

ARM: A Real-Time Health Monitoring Mobile Application

Saeid Pourroostaei Ardakani$^{(\boxtimes)}$ ⓘ, Xuting Wu, Shuning Pan, and Xinyu Gao

School of Computer Science, University of Nottingham Ningbo China,
Ningbo 315100, China
{saeid.ardakani,scyxw1,zy22054,scyxg1}@nottingham.edu.cn

Abstract. Considering the risks and difficulties of providing in-patient medical services, this is of great significance to develop mobile applications which are able to provide remote healthcare. This paper proposes a Real-time Health Monitoring Mobile Application that enables patients to remotely report health cues to healthcare teams and receive treatment plans. This allows healthcare team to collect and analyse blood oxygen, heart rate and body temperature which are reported by a Bluetooth interconnected sensory device. Yet, a chat environment is provided that allows patients to submit self-questionaries and communicate with healthcare teams in real time. In addition, this allows healthcare teams to access the patients' health records and profiles and remotely monitor their health status. According to the test results (i.e., functional, system, front-end, back-end and hardware), this mobile application is able to offer a number of promising benefits -mainly remote basic checkup with minimum contact risks especially during COVID-19 pandemic.

Keywords: Wearable sensors · Remote sensing · Healthcare · Mobile communications

1 Introduction

Recent advances and innovations in accessibility and usability of mobile devices and wearables form a new life style. Smartphones can be used almost everywhere and provide users required services including education, healthcare, marketing and logistics. Users stay connected and access to a wide range of information, applications and services as required. Healthcare is one of the key fields that benefits from mobile and digital technologies by interconnecting healthcare stacksholders beyond time and geographical location [1].

Mobile health (M-health) [2] applications offer a number of benefits such as resource conservation, treatment compliance enhancement and healthcare service accessibility improvement to healthcare stakeholders. According to [3], m-health has the potential to significantly reduce healthcare cost and enhance patient convenience. For example, M-health applications provide patients remote consultation and health check-up that results in reduced treatment cost and time [4].

© ICST Institute for Computer Sciences, Social Informatics and Telecommunications Engineering 2021
Published by Springer Nature Switzerland AG 2021. All Rights Reserved
J. A. Marmolejo-Saucedo et al. (Eds.): COMPSE 2021, LNICST 393, pp. 45–59, 2021.
https://doi.org/10.1007/978-3-030-87495-7_4

In-patient treatments, particularly, are usually expensive and resource consuming (e.g. time) as patients need to visit hospitals to receive healthcare services. As [5] outlines, in-patient healthcare is one of the largest expenditures, about one trillion USD in the United States. Hence, researchers and scientists are highly interested in proposing and utilising M-health applications to reduce healthcare risk, decrease cost and conserve healthcare resources especially during COVID-19 pandemic where healthcare resources are restricted and in-patient treatment is highly risk-full.

This article proposes a real-time health monitoring mobile application (ARM) through which healthcare teams would be able to remotely monitor patients and provide them required treatment instructions with minimum physical contact. Indeed, the target is to improve healthcare treatment efficiency and enhance convenience. Patients fill out online healthcare questionnaires and utilise wearable sensors to report body data such as heartbeat, blood oxygen and body temperature. Health records are forwarded to the healthcare team for further monitoring and treatment planning after the patients' profile is updated. In addition, ARM provides a chat channel through which healthcare teams and patients would be able to communicate in real time.

ARM has the capacity of providing mobile healthcare services. By this, healthcare teams would be able to remotely monitor patients, communicate to observe basic disease signs and plan the required treatments. During the pandemic peak, it is repeatedly announced by the health organisations that people should avoid visiting clinic for simple/basic diseases such as flu. Patients are asked to wear masks if they urgently need to visit their GPs. Although wearing masks could slow down the spreading speed of the virus, this could not be assumed as a long-term solution to manage the virus outbreak. Healthcare technologies (e.g. M-health) are promising approaches to solve this problem as they can reduce physical contact. Moreover, they are able to conserve resources -mainly time and expense [6]. For example, it roughly takes 30 min to collect temperature, blood pressure, heart rate, height and weight information for each in-patient visit. Long queues and increased waiting time are unbearable especially when the healthcare services are restricted (e.g. during COVID-19 pandemic) and/or patients are under pain (e.g. stomachache). ARM tackles these issues by allowing healthcare teams to remotely collect patients' basic health data.

This paper is organised as follows: Sect. 2 reviews literatures and outlines M-health applications and technologies. Section 3 introduces ARM and explains design, implementation features and techniques. Section 4 discusses testing results to highlight this mobile application's achievements. Section 5 concludes ARM benefits and outlines the key points of future work.

2   Related Work

There are a number of M-health applications in the market providing users healthcare data collection, communication and monitoring services. However, they still suffer from key drawbacks -mainly online communication and lack of real-time body data collection and analysis. Yet, some of the mobile applications are dedicatedly designed for specific diseases or particular applications.

LabVIEW [7] proposes a healthcare mobile application that measures user's physical data by using wearable sensors to monitor health fitness. In addition, this system alarms users via text/email in the case of health risk or hazard. However, this provides users no communication, feedback or interaction to approach healthcare teams.

[8] introduces a mobile healthcare application dedicatedly designed for diabetes patients. This platform is interconnected to Electronic Medical Record (EMR) system to report and collect patients' records. It analyses the latest patient's blood sugar records which are reported by EMR and offers the patients treatment plans.

BiliCam [9] proposes a mobile application through which newborn jaundice can be detected and reported. For this, smartphone's camera scans infant's skin and the image result is compared with a colour sample card. It extracts the skin colour features and detects how close the skin colour is to the samples, which diagnoses the level of jaundice. Yet, a machine learning technique is used to train datasets and optimise the results. HemaApp [10] is another mobile application that utilises smartphone's camera to measure haemoglobin levels using a similar technique.

[11] focuses on a mobile application that collects and reports behaviours of patients with Schizophrenia. For this, smartphone's accelerometer, microphone and global positioning system are used to collect patients' location, activity and speech during daily life. This provides patients fitted feedback according to their collected behaviour.

Seismo [12] presents a smartphone application through which blood pressure is collected and monitored. For this, smartphone accelerometer and camera report the heart vibration and pulse from the user's fingerprint. By this, the user is able to monitor blood pressure if any treatment is required.

[13] proposes a mobile application design and implementation that is used to monitor physical activity for patients with chronic heart-failure in real time. It utilises smart-phone's embedded sensors to collect body data and forwards them for an off-line analysis.

ClinTouch [14] focuses on a M-health mobile application which is designed for mental issues and diseases. This is implemented and evaluated as a pilot to provide symptom tracker, diary function and appointment reminder services. However, it matches no National Health Service (NHS) principals due to the lack of solid safety and security.

[15] proposes a mobile application which provides doctor-patient real-time communication. However, it supports no data collection of patients and remote healthcare monitoring.

ARM aims to combine the key healthcare features to propose a mobile application which is able to manage healthcare records and treatment plans, collect body data with minimum physical contact and provide real-time communication with doctors. According to the literature, it is learned that existing mobile applications lack such combination to provide healthcare services if real-time communication, on-demand data collection and online monitoring are required.

3   The Proposed Approach

This section introduces a healthcare mobile application that allows patients and healthcare teams are kept interconnected. By this, body data, such as body temperature, blood oxygen and heart rate is collected and reported to healthcare teams for further analysis and utilisation. This M-health mobile application is able to automatically report patients' health status using a sensory platform and online questionnaire. In addition, this allows patients and healthcare teams to manage their profiles and provides them personalised healthcare applications. Yet, this allows the healthcare stakeholders to communicate and supports real-time feedback through an interactive social environment.

Android Studio (3.5.3) is used to implement the mobile application platform as this supports portability and utility. Android is a well-known open-source, flexible and adaptable programming platform that is widely used to implement mobile applications [16]. Yet, this version of android studio supports several permission protocols including internet and WRITE_EXTERNAL_STORAGE that are usually used to provide security and user privacy. This allows users to access information once required permissions are granted.

ARM is implemented by Java to support portability and cross-functionality on desktops, mobiles and/or embedded systems. Java is object-oriented, therefore codes are easy to extend and fix. Java supports multithreading and network computation and provides multimedia. Besides, this enhances project development by separating the characteristics using object-oriented programming.

The proposed system is designed as three components including sensory module, core application and database. The Sensory module stays on the duty of body area data collection including blood oxygen, heart rate and temperature. The Core application is responsible for data analysis. This utilises body data from the Bluetooth-connected sensory module to offer healthcare functions. If some body data is out of the normal range, a message with automatic diagnosis and abnormal data will be sent to both the user and the healthcare team. Database component manages the collected data to response to either user or healthcare team enquires. Figure 1 depicts ARM conceptual diagram.

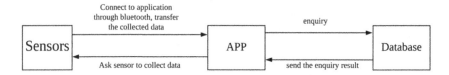

Fig. 1. ARM system architecture.

ARM's Core Application. The core application is designed and set-up for both stakeholders including doctor and patient. As Fig. 2 shows, users need to register and fill out a questionnaire to access the mobile application. There are three major functions: HOME, CHAT and MY page. HOME allows patients to make a health appointment, visit a doctor online, observe health report and monitor the treatment process. Healthcare teams use HOME to check patients' information and give them treatment/advice. CHAT is also available for both patients and healthcare teams when they need to communicate in real-time by using text messages. Yet, MY page allows the users to update profiles, set-up sensory communication through Bluetooth, view history records and log out of the system.

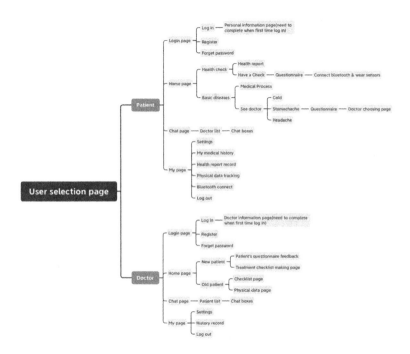

Fig. 2. ARM's Core Application Chart.

According to Fig. 3, ARM's sequence diagram outlines how the users interact with the system from a patient's perspective. By this, first, the patient chooses a disease type and waits until the system returns a questionnaire focusing on the disease to collect data. ARM provides a list of registered doctors with their availability hours/days once the patient submits the questionnaire. This forwards the questionnaire data to the doctor as this is selected. The corresponding doctor makes a treatment checklist and sends this back to the patient to collect the required information -mainly body area data such as temperature, blood oxygen and heart rate. Yet, the patient and doctor are kept interconnected to monitor the treatment procedure until good results are achieved.

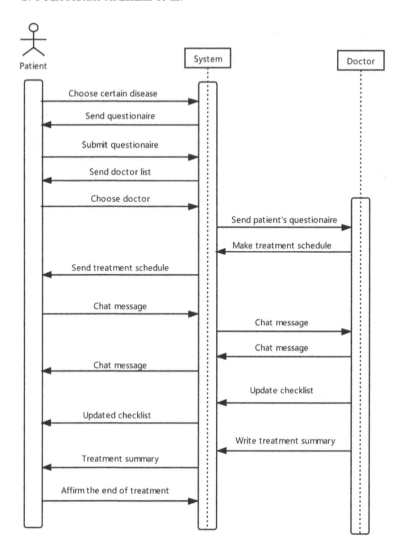

Fig. 3. ARM's sequence diagram.

ARM's Sensory Module. ARM's sensory module is set-up to collect and forward body area data. As Fig. 4 shows, this is comprised of three parts: sensors, Arduino mini controller and Bluetooth. MH-ET LIVE_MAX30102 Arduino chip [17] is used for body area data collection. This integrates a body temperature sensor, heart rate sensor and blood oxygen sensor. This is a small and easy to set- up sensor with a size of $(2\,cm \times 1\,cm \times 1\,mm)$. Arduino board MEGA 2560 [18] is a micro-controller that is interconnected to the MAX30102 sensory device. This is able to process data -mainly in-aggregation and transmit information through various communication technologies, such as Bluetooth, USB,

GSM and I2C. ARM utilises Bluetooth to provide a communication tie between MEGA 2560 and MAX30102. The reason to choose this technology is that Bluetooth reduces costs as compared to infrastructure-based networks -mainly GSM. MEGA 2560 board is programmed using Arduino studio in C programming language. Arduino studio provides many useful functions and libraries, such as serial port monitoring and drawing.

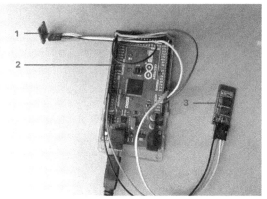

1. Sensor-MH-ET LIVE _MAX30102

2. Arduino Mini Controller (MEGA-2560)

3. Bluetooth -HC-05

Fig. 4. ARM's sensory module.

ARM's Database Design. ARM database conceptual diagram is depicted as Fig. 5. According to this, DoctorAccount, DoctorBasicInformation, PatientAccount, PatientBasicInformation are the key database tables that store the user information for both doctors and patients. Each user is provided by a particular user account (DoctorAccount and PatientAccount) which updates user profile information. Yet, doctors' and patients' basic information including name, speciality, degree, age and gender is stored in DoctorBasicInformation and PatientBasicInformation respectively. In addition, doctor-patient communication information such as date and title are recorded at the ChattingMessage table. This would help the healthcare teams to re-consider past appointments and patients' healthcare records. Patient_Questionnaire keeps the questionnaire information which is provided by the patients regarding the health issue. This returns the patient's health self-report which can be used by doctors to figure out the health issue and/or disease. DoctorTimetable provides the doctor availability time-slots and is used to show the list of available appointments.

HealthCheckRecord table records the results of health checkups and/or treatments according to the appointment given by AppointmentList. Then, a checklist (CheckList table) is provided for patient patients to update their healthcare records accordingly. FinishAppointment is used to record the appointment timing values and keep the start and end times of the treatment.

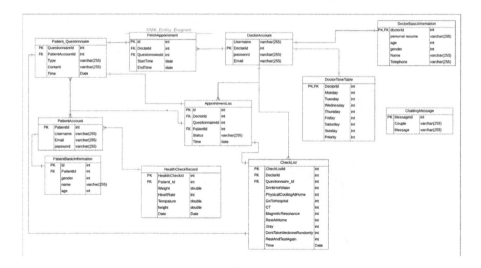

Fig. 5. ARM's Database design.

4   Results and Discussions

The proposed android application aims to provide remote monitoring/treatment, patient/doctor interconnection and body area data collection. Figure 6 shows ARM's user interface. To evaluate ARM's performance, comprehensive testing is conducted for functional, system, front-end, back-end and hardware testing.

Functional Testing. Functional testing aims to check whether ARM is able to perform the designed operations or not. However, ARM is not tested by real patients and doctors. Non-professional users (e.g., students) used this app to test its functionality. It can be addressed as future work to test this app by professional users such as healthcare teams.

Functional testing is conducted to test the following operations as Table 1. According to the test plan and achieved results, the following responses are recorded for each particular test operation/scenario.

System Testing. System testing focuses on system recovery which aims to check how ARM is able to recover in the case of any crash or hardware failure. For this, a hardware crash is simulated through a shut-down mechanism using which ARM server is suddenly re-started and the database is re-built. This evaluates ARM performance and database recovery in the case of a server crash. A registration operation is used to test the system's functionality. By this, the database should be able to successfully retrieve the registration information if the system is re-started after a sudden shut down (or crash).

To evaluate system scalability, ARM functionality is tested when multiple users simultaneously log in. For this, a test scenario is designed through which

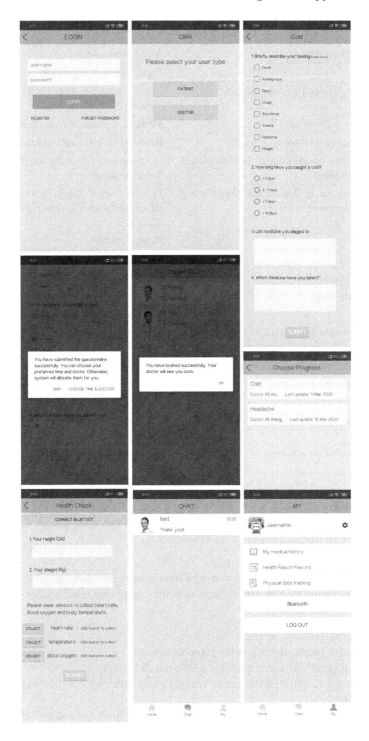

Fig. 6. ARM's UI.

Table 1. Functional test plan and results

Test operation/scenario	ARM response
Register	Verification code is sent
Log in 1) registered 2) unregistered	1) User's profile appears 2) Ask to register
View medical progress	Medical records are displayed
Patient chooses disease (e.g. cold)	Forward to relevant questionnaire
Filling out the questionnaire 1) Completed 2) Uncompleted	1) Questionnaire submitted 2) Error message
Choosing doctor 1) Automatic allocation 2) Manual allocation	1) Free doctor is automatically allocated 2) the selected doctor is allocated
Health history	Health profile
Have a check	Health check page
Bluetooth connection	Connect to Bluetooth
Collect body data	Sensor measures and reports
Tracking	View health records
Update personal information: 1) True information 2) Wrong information	1) Successful updated 2) Error
Doctor visits patients 1) New 2) Existing	1) New profile 2) Past records
Doctor monitors patient	Updated patient's records
Doctor provides feedback	Feedback form filled out
Doctor edits questionnaire/checklist as required	Questionnaire updated
Real-time communication	Private text-chat room

60 test users try to work with ARM at the same time for 10 min as a simple check-up. During the testing period, no obvious delay and system failure was detected and all operations went on smoothly.

Front-End Testing. Front-end testing focuses on evaluating the Graphical user interface, functionality and application usability. The test results are outlined as below:

- All designed buttons work.
- All designed pages are correctly interconnected.
- Layouts appear the same as what has been designed.
- User receives alarm "Please enter correct email address" if the email address is not valid.
- User receives alarm "Username and password cannot be empty" if any field of the user account is left empty.

- User receives alarm 'Passwords are inconsistent' if 'Password' and 'Confirm Password' are different.
- User cannot enter letters in fields that only accept numbers like 'Height' and 'Weight'.

Back-End Testing. Back-end testing examines whether the system is able to correctly respond the user requests or not. This is conducted as follows: one test user, android phone ARM, the corresponding sensors and the database server. By this, the user submits a number of new transactions to modify database records. The objective is to study how the ARM database is dealt with the new transactions according to the system requirements. Table 2 summarises back-end results for each operation which is designed according to the testing scenario.

Table 2. Back-end testing results

Test operation	ARM response	Database response
Mismatched username and password	Error	Username and password not exists
Update profile	Update message	Database record is updated
Submit questionnaire	Submission message	Database record is updated
Wrong checklist/question provided	Error	No database update

Hardware Testing. Hardware testing evaluates system functionality, sensory device stability, system/sensor compatibility and measurement error rate. Hardware testing results are outlined as below:

System Functionality

- If the users frequently move their fingers or wrongly use the sensor, data collection fails or returns inaccurate results.

Sensory Device Stability

- Particular factors (e.g. weather and skin sweat) may address wrong results.
- Users may lose their patience while data collection as this requires to have 10 s finger-touch to collect multiple sensory data.

System/sensor Compatibility

- ARM bluetooth connection may fail if any other application is used during the Bluetooth connection.
- ARM can't read sensory data if Bluetooth is not successfully interconnected.

Table 3. The comparison of ARM with the literatures

Features	ARM	LabVIEW [7]	[8]	BiliCam [9]	HemaApp [10]	[11]	Seismo [12]	ClinTouch [14]	[15]
Real-time health data collection/analysis	Y	Y	N	Y	Y	Y	Y	Y	N
Body data collection	Y	Y	N	Y	Y	Y	Y	N	N
(Offline) Communication	Y	Y	Y	Y	Y	Y	Y	Y	N
Realtime chat	Y	N	N	Y	Y	Y	N	Y	Y
User profile	Y	N	Y	N	N	N	Y	Y	Y
Healthcare Service management	Y	N	Y	N	N	N	Y	Y	Y
Multi-functionality	Y	Y	N	N	N	Y	Y	Y	Y

Measurement Error Rate

– The accuracy of the measurements is about 92%. This calculates as 55 out of 60 test users correctly report the sensory data.

5   Conclusion and Further Work

ARM is comprised of three key modules questionnaire, chatting environment, and sensory design. The questionnaire are designed to collect health self-report from the patients. For this, the questions are designed according to the user health issues and data requirement. For example, a patient who suffers from stomach should be provided a questionnaire which asks for stomach symptoms and required data collection. For this, doctors, specialists and healthcare teams would select/design the required questions from a questionnaire checklist to collect the required information from the patients. Indeed, the designed questionnaires should be able to capture key information of patients' symptoms and health issues. Chatting module is used to make a real-time communication between the healthcare team and patients. This allows both user-sides to share additional required data and/or discuss about the treatment plan. This allows the patients to report their uncommon symptoms or disease signs which are not covered by the provided questionnaire. Sensor design is used to collect body area data. This allows doctors to remotely collect patients body data with no physical interaction. This allows doctors to use accurate and realtime data to investigate the health issue and plan the required treatment.

ARM provides online health monitoring that offers a number of benefits to enhance the quality of healthcare services. This aims to keep patients and healthcare teams interconnected and collect and analyse physiological data in real-time. ARM's remote and real-time body data collection/analysis would result in reduction of healthcare monitoring cost and risk especially during COVID-19 pandemic. ARM is multi-functional which has the potential to be utilised for various healthcare scenarios and applications. This provides real-time links for healthcare stockholders (doctors and patients) to communicate through. Yet, ARM allows the users to create and update their profiles. Patients' profiles are linked to the healthcare records which can be accessed by the doctors during treatment procedures, whereas doctor's profiles provide their updated experiences, availabilities and specialities. Moreover, ARM allows healthcare teams to manage/schedule healthcare services and inform the patients online. Table 3 summarises the advantages of ARM as compared with the literatures.

To evaluate ARM performance, five test plans are conducted: functional, system, front-end, back-end, and hardware testing. The results of functional testing shows that ARM is able to manage the user transactions in general. System testing results show that ARM is scalable and able to manage multiple simultaneous. Moreover, this has the capacity of full system recovery in the case of sudden hardware crash. Front-end testing supports that ARM user interface is fully implemented and correctly work. Back-end testing shows that ARM is able to manage data records and correctly forward and reply database transactions and queries. Hardware testing results study the influence of hardware factors on sensory data collection and communication. This shows that the accuracy and reliability of collected body data, disease recognition and treatment plan is highly dependent on the hardware factors.

There are three issues that can be addressed as further work. First, to enhance the functionality and operation of ARM's chat environment. The chat environment supports only text communication which is comparatively restricted. For this, providing audio/video communication between the doctors and patients would be a new feature which allows them to communicate easier and more convenience. Second, a chatbot can be designed to improve ARM functionality and user-friendly. This chatbot should be able to automatically recognise the user's questions and provide them relevant answer and/or help/signpost them to find the required information. Text mining approaches should be used to recognise the keywords and link them into the answer pools. Yet, machine learning techniques are required to continuously update the answers based on users' feedback. According to [19], the chatbot can be fed by key healthcare information centres and/or key references to provide best-fitted answers based on the user's questions. With the help of collected sensor data and the context of user input, the implementation of machining learning algorithm and clinical decision-making helps users obtain their expected answers quickly. If the patients are satisfied with the automatically generated answers, they could choose to stop the service thus save both patients and doctors time. Third, this is required to consult with COVID-19 pandemic specialists to re-design this application dedicatedly for COVID-19. During COVID-19 pandemic, this is very risky for patients to visit hospitals and clinics in person [20]. For this, ARM would be able to offer a number of benefits such as patients distance monitoring, remote treatment which reduces the outbreak and conserve the resources. Indeed, ARM would be able to recognise COVID-19 symptoms (e.g. such as cough, fatigue and diarrhoea) and provide required treatment plans with minimum physical contact between doctors and patients.

References

1. Mariakakis, A., Wang, E., Goel, M., Patel, S.: Challenges in realizing smartphone-based health sensing. IEEE Pervasive Comput. **18**(2), 76–84 (2019)
2. World Health Organization: mhealth: new horizons for health through mobile technologies: based on the findings of the second global survey on ehealth (2019). https://www.who.int/goe/publications/goemhealthweb.pdf. Accessed Jan 2020
3. Banga, B.: Global mobile medical apps market to reach usd11.22 billion by 2025, reports BIS research (2020). https://www.prnewswire.com/news-releases/. Accessed Aug 2020
4. Cosco, T.D., Firth, J., Vahia, I., Sixsmith, A., Torous, J.: Mobilizing mhealth data collection in older adults: challenges and opportunities. JMIR Aging **2**(1), 1–8 (2019)
5. Elflein, J.: Hospital care expenditure in the united states from 1960 to 2020 (2020). https://www.statista.com/statistics/184772/us-hospital-care-expenditures-since-1960/. Accessed July 2020
6. Hanrahan, C., Aungst, T.D., Cole, S.: Evaluating mobile medical applications. American Society of Health-System Pharmacists Inc., Technical report (2014)
7. Abdullah, A., Ismael, A., Rashid, A., Abou-ElNour, A., Tarique, M.: Real time wireless health monitoring application using mobile devices. Int. J. Comput. Netw. Commun. **7**(3), 13–30 (2015)
8. Jung, E.Y., Kim, J., Chung, K.Y., Park, D.K.: Mobile healthcare application with EMR interoperability for diabetes patients. Clust. Comput. **17**(3), 871–880 (2013)
9. de Greef, L., et al.: BiliCam: using mobile phones to monitor newborn jaundice. In: ACM International Joint Conference on Pervasive and Ubiquitous Computing (UbiComp 2014), Seattle, Washington, US, 13–17 September 2014 (2014)
10. Wang, E.J., Zhu, W.L.J., Rana, R., Patel, S.N.: Noninvasive hemoglobin measurement using unmodified smartphone camera and white flash. In: 39th Annual International Conference of the IEEE Engineering in Medicine and Biology Society (EMBC), Seogwipo, South Korea, 11–15 July 2017 (2017)
11. Ben-Zeev, D., et al.: Mobile behavioral sensing for outpatients and inpatients with schizophrenia. Psychiatr. Serv. (Washington, D.C.) **67**(5), 557–561 (2016)
12. Wang, E.J., et al.: Seismo: blood pressure monitoring using built-in smartphone accelerometer and camera. In: ACM Conference on Human-Computer Interaction (CHI 2018), Montreal, QC, Canada, 21–26 April 2018 (2018)
13. Aranki, D., Kurillo, G., Yan, P., Liebovitz, D.M., Bajcsy, R.: Real-time tele-monitoring of patients with chronic heart-failure using a smartphone: lessons learned. IEEE Trans. Affect. Comput. **7**(3), 206–219 (2016)
14. Hollis, C., et al.: Technological innovations in mental healthcare: harnessing the digital revolution. Br. J. Psychiatry **206**(4), 263–265 (2015)
15. Nwabueze, E.E., Oju, O.: Using mobile application to improve doctor-patient interaction in healthcare delivery system. E-Health Telecommun. Syst. Netw. **8**(3), 23–34 (2019)
16. Shah, K.: How benefits of android app can help businesses (2019). https://www.rishabhsoft.com/blog/5-advantages-of-android-app-development-for-your-business. Accessed May 2020

17. Maxim Integrated: High-sensitivity pulse oximeter and heart-rate sensor for wearable health (2020). https://www.maximintegrated.com/en/products/interface/sensor-interface/MAX30102.html. Accessed Jan 2020
18. Arduino: Arduino mega 2560 and genuino mega 2560 (2020). https://www.arduino.cc/en/pmwiki.php?n=Main/ArduinoBoardMega2560. Accessed Jan 2020
19. Divya, S., Indumathi, V., Ishwarya, S., Priyasankari, M., Devi, S.K.: A self-diagnosis medical chatbot using artificial intelligence. J. Web Dev. Web Design. **3**(1), 1–7 (2018)
20. Centers for Disease Control and Prevention: People with certain medical conditions (2020). https://www.cdc.gov/coronavirus/2019-ncov/need-extra-precautions/people-with-medical-conditions.html. Accessed Sept 2020

Computer and Data Science

Network Coding and Dispersal Information with TCP for Content Delivery

Francisco de Asís López-Fuentes[1]($\boxtimes$), Raúl Antonio Ortega-Vallejo[1], and Ricardo Marcelín-Jiménez[2]

[1] Universidad Autónoma Metropolitana-Cuajimalpa, Av. Vasco de Quiroga 4871, Cuajimalpa, 05348 Mexico City, Mexico
flopez@cua.uam.mx, raulantonio@protonmail.com
[2] Universidad Autónoma Metropolitana-Iztapalapa, Av. Atlixco 186, Iztapalapa, 09340 Mexico City, Mexico
cal@xanum.uam.mx

Abstract. Dissemination information from many sources to many receivers can be fundamental in different systems. However, the components of these system may present some failure type both the software and hardware. In addition, problems related to the communication networks such as limited bandwidth or packet loss should be present. The information dispersal algorithm (IDA) has been used as a good solution to offer fault tolerance. On the other hand, network coding is a coding method mainly used to increase throughput of a communication channel, which is useful to face the limited bandwidth in the communication networks. In this paper, we integrate both methods into a content distribution scheme. We use a hybrid peer-to-peer (P2P) network based on TCP in order to evaluate the performance of IDA and network coding in a joint operation.

Keywords: Network coding · Information dispersal · P2P networks · TCP

1 Introduction

Content delivery is very popular today, users can exchange several content types such as video, text messages, PDF documents, music, and photos. Some content such as video demand for a large amount of resources from the Internet infrastructures and cooperation between nodes play an important role. New problems such as fault tolerance, limited performance or bandwidth limitations have emerged. To face these challenges some techniques such as the information dispersal algorithm (IDA) [1] and network coding [2] have been proposed. Using IDA in the communication systems we can reach redundancy of the information in different levels and make better use of the storage capacities of the devices. In this way, we can configure fault-tolerance storage systems more efficient. On the other hand, network coding allows that the intermediate nodes encode the received packets for immediately forwarding the encoded packets to the end nodes [3, 4] and [5]. In other words, the packets received in the intermediate nodes are combined before

© ICST Institute for Computer Sciences, Social Informatics and Telecommunications Engineering 2021
Published by Springer Nature Switzerland AG 2021. All Rights Reserved
J. A. Marmolejo-Saucedo et al. (Eds.): COMPSE 2021, LNICST 393, pp. 63–72, 2021.
https://doi.org/10.1007/978-3-030-87495-7_5

forwarding them to the following nodes. Network coding uses elements of a finite field for the linear operations during the packet manipulation. The communications systems can be benefited by using network coding because this technique helps to increase the throughput and reduce the latency. Although different benefits by using network coding and IDA are reported in the literature [18, 19], both techniques have been used separately. This paper proposes an architecture where the IDA and network coding are combined. Peers are used as a way to improve the content delivery. Our proposed architecture is implemented using TCP. We use specific characteristics of this protocol such as the retransmission as a way to reduce the number of descriptors to be sent to each intermediate node.

This paper has the following organization. Section 2 presents related work to IDA and network coding. Section 3 introduces basic and fundamental aspects of network coding and IDA. In this section, we also explain some concepts about P2P networks and TCP. Section 4 presents our proposed architecture, where network coding and the information dispersal algorithm are combined under TCP. Our implementation and an initial evaluation is described in Sect. 5. Our conclusions are presented in Sect. 6.

2 Related Work

Several studies to address the impact of redundancy on P2P storage systems have been reported in the scientific community. Many of these works have related with network coding and the information dispersal algorithm (IDA). The works of [10, 11, and 12] evaluate redundancy assuming a static network. In [10], there is a thorough analytical study of the mean-time to failure (MTTF), bandwidth and storage load, for either simple replication or error-codes, particularly based on Rabin's IDA [1]. Failures on the set of storage devices are regarded as independent and identically distributed (iid) random variables. The main result shows that, compared to simple replication, IDA provides by far a higher MTTF, under the same amount of redundancy. Also, IDA requires less bandwidth and storage. In turn, [11] is focused on the excess of information required to different strategies, in order to provide the same level of availability for a collection of files. This study is based on Monte-Carlo simulations. Each experiment consists of a number of files which are processed according to a given strategy, and require allocation on the devices that make up the system. Nevertheless, devices are available with a given probability. The main result here is that IDA needs less space to provide the same level of availability, compared to simple replication. The second part of [11], is an effort to consider the long term behavior of a P2P storage network. For this purpose, any peer connection is assumed to last an exponential random time. The findings show that the files' availability presents a faster degradation when stored under IDA replication. In [12], the study compares three strategies: *uncoded random storage, traditional erasure coding based storage, and random linear coding based storage.* The result proposes that network codes are a good option to maintain the best efficiency of the system. Two important studies [13, 14] developed models that evaluate the amount of redundant information delivered by either simple replication or IDA, according to the level of availability required by the set of allocated files. Also, both works addressed the problem of maintainability, i.e. the cost of recovering and reallocating the information stored in a peer which is presumed to be left permanently. They introduced the concept of membership expiration time, in order to estimate whether a disconnection should be regarded as temporal or permanent. Using this parameter they developed a formula to evaluate the amount of average peer bandwidth required to keep any file within a given level of availability. Apart from simple replication, IDA and the hybrid approach by [13], the work of [15] introduces network codes. The study is based on analytical models and trace-driven simulations. Their findings show that network codes provide a very efficient mechanism to support information maintenance. Authors in [18] use IDA to make an efficient content delivery on a P2P network. A solution for a secure PLC (Power Line Communication) communication among end nodes based on the Information Dispersal Algorithm (IDA) is presented in [20]. In this work, the authors propose an efficient scheme using the physical characteristics of PLC channels of a smart grid.

On the other hand, network coding have used in several works for content delivery, because this technique has already proven to provide solutions to a variety of networking problems. For example, authors in [16] presents a unified linear program formulation for optimal content delivery in content delivery networks (CDNs). In this work, different costs and constraints associated with content disseminations are considered from the source node to storage nodes. The end users can do an eventual fetching of content of storage nodes. In [17] network coding is deployed in the backbone network for an IPTV architecture. In this case, network coding helps to increase network capacity while improving robustness against network faults. Authors in [21] introduce ND-POR, which is a scheme based on network coding but it is observed that these can be sensitive to a certain type of small corruption attack on their integrity and, to turn it around, the dispersal coding is applied. This proposal has the main target the cloud storage systems. To the best of our knowledge, in most of the literature reviewed, both network coding and IDA have been used separately. In this paper is presented a collaborative architecture which combines network coding and IDA with TCP over a hybrid P2P network in order to evaluate the performance of both technique during content delivery. Peers help to improve the packets delivery, while TCP allows to reduce the number of descriptors to be sent to the intermediate nodes.

3   Background

Information redundancy is an important concern of any communication system. This important characteristic can be reached via replication or coding. However, both techniques have different approach. For example, using replication we can allocate 3 copies of a file F, on 3 different storage sites. In this way, a failure in 2 storage sites can be tolerated by the system. Nevertheless, the effective storage capacity is only one third of the overall capacity. Now, we review information redundancy using IDA [1]. In this case, file F is transformed into n dispersals, each one of size $|F|/m$ and F can be recovered provided that any m out of n dispersals remain available (see Fig. 1). We can see in Fig. 2 that it is only required n/m × 100% of the original file size as redundant information using IDA. Let us suppose that we use a particular implementation of IDA with parameters n = 5, and m = 3. Compared to the previous case of replication, the file can be transformed into n = 5 dispersal, each of size $|F|/3$. In this case is produced an excess of information of $(5/3) \times 100\%$, which is less than 300% of information required by the replication strategy. Thus, any 2 dispersals can be loosed, but it is still possible to recover the original file. Based on this approach, IDA presents an effective capacity almost twice compared with the replication strategy. This scenario is shown in Fig. 2.

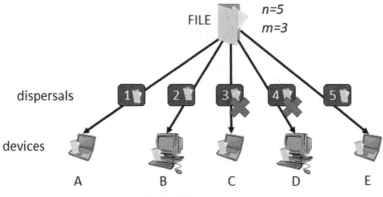

Fig. 1. IDA concept.

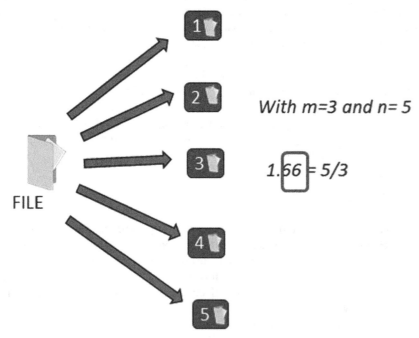

Fig. 2. An example of IDA for m = 3 and n = 5.

Network coding is an encoding technique used to increase the flow of packets without exceeding the link capacity [2]. To explain this scenario, we use a butterfly network (see

Fig. 3), which has a source node S, and two receiving nodes R1 and R2. Each edge has capacity of 1 as shown in Fig. 3a, and we can see that the maximum flow from the source S to any receiver (R1 or R2) has a value of 2. Simultaneously, source S sends bit b1 to receiver R1 and bit b2 to R2 (see Fig. 3b). Node 3 receives bits b1 and b2 from nodes 1 and 2, respectively, and it must send both bits to node 4. However, the link between nodes 3 and 4 requires two time units to send both bits. In contrast, using network coding (which is indicated with the operator ⊕ in Fig. 3c) the receiver R1 can recover both bits (b1 and b2), but bit b2 must be recovered from operation b1 ⊕ b2. Receiver R2 recovers both bits making a similar procedure as R1. In this scenario, node 3 is responsible to apply network coding. We can note that network coding allows to increase the multicast rate in the link from 1 to 2 bits/time unit.

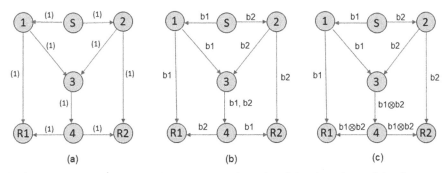

Fig. 3. Example of a communication network. a) Capacity of the edges, b) Traditional approach and c) approach with network coding.

P2P networks have become a popular paradigm for the next generation of distributed computing, and they are used to spread digital content to a large audience [6]. These types of networks are a research topic in several areas such as data communication networks, distributed systems, complexity theory and databases [7]. A P2P network is a virtual communication infrastructure deployed over a physical network. Nodes build a network abstraction on top of the physical network, and it is known as an overlay network. This overlay network is independent of the underlying physical network, and the connections between nodes are done using the Transmission Control Protocol (TCP). This protocol allows to abstract the physical connections in such a way that these are not reflected in the overlay network. The routing mechanisms use the logical tunnels implemented between nodes by the overlay network [8]. TCP is a transport protocol used to provide reliable delivery of data via a communication network [9]. Computers can exchange data with application programs in a way correct, secure and in order by using TCP. Communication networks can present packet loss during a transmission. To deal with this problem TCP uses retransmission to ensure the delivery of the packets. TCP can do n number of retransmissions, depending on the number of lost packets during the transmission. In this work, we combine IDA and network coding using TCP over a P2P infrastructure.

4   Proposed Model

This section describes our proposed model. Figure 4 shows our architecture, which is formed by 15 different nodes (peers and servers).

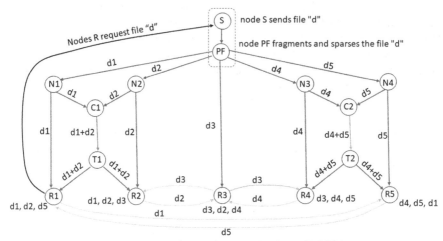

Fig. 4. Architecture combining network coding and IDA.

Node S is the source node, while node PF is the fragmenting peer, which is the responsible to fragment the file using the information dispersal algorithm (IDA). We use two butterfly schemes to deploy network coding. The nodes N1 and N2 are the source nodes in the butterfly 1, while N3 and N4 are the source nodes in the butterfly 2. Nodes C1 and C2 are the intermediate nodes which are responsible to do the network coding operation in the butterfly 1 and 2, respectively. Node T1 relays the encoded message received from the node C1 to the requesting nodes R1 and R2 in the butterfly 1, while node T2 relays the encoded message received from the node C2 to the requesting nodes R4 and R5 in the butterfly 2. The requesting peer R3 receives the descriptor from the node PF directly. All requesting nodes R are working as peers, which establish communication between them to share the descriptors and to have information about the contents that are shared within the network. For each delivery, a peer R creates a thread to distribute the received descriptor to other peers. The communication between a sending peer and a requesting peer is established through this thread. All nodes in the architecture have a specific role during the transmission, therefore they are renamed before that a file be sent to a requesting peer. All peers (nodes R) collaborate with each other to distribute a descriptor in our architecture. That is to say, the peers work as relay node too. This means that a peer receives a dispersal from the fragmenting node (PF) or node T and retransmits this dispersal to other peers in the architecture. For example, node R3 receives descriptor d3 from node PF, then d3 is relayed to nodes R2 and R4. On the other hand, node R1 receives descriptor d1 from node N1, then d1 is relayed to node R5. Nodes R2, R4 and

R5 have a similar behavior as node R1 because they only distribute a descriptor. Our proposed architecture works as a multi-source scheme because the nodes R receive three different dispersals from three different nodes.

Initially, the source sends the requested file by the requesting nodes R to the fragmenting node, which uses the IDA algorithm to fragment the file into five descriptors. Each receiver node R can recover the original file having only three descriptors. The fragmenting node requests the IP addresses of the nodes (N1, N2, R3, N3 and N4). Each of these IP addresses receives a descriptor from The PF node. After this, nodes N work as sources, and network coding is applied using two butterfly schemes. Nodes R1, R2, R4 and R5 recover two descriptors by decoding the message received from the nodes T. These receiving nodes with two descriptors establish communication with the other requesting nodes to delivery their descriptors. Because node R3 only receives a descriptor, this node should receive a descriptor from nodes R2 and R4. Thus, all requesting nodes R obtain the missing descriptor and they can assemble the original file using the IDA algorithm.

5 Implementation and Evaluation

Our work is in progress, and we have done an initial implementation of our architecture. This prototype has been developed in the C programming language for the Debian Linux operating system. Our prototype uses 14 containers and we performed 6 runs for each experiment. We transmitted different source vectors with the following dimensions: 1 MB, 5 MB, 10 MB, 15 MB, and 30 MB.

Our first experiment evaluates a content delivery using IDA without network coding. In this case, the butterflies are not done, and the nodes R receive the descriptors directly from the nodes N. Thus, the most intensive interaction occurs between the R nodes and the nodes N, which must retransmit the flow from the node PF. Nodes N work as relay nodes. Each vector is simulated as a broadcast, where because TCP is used. The nodes N require concurrent processes to emit a vector "d". The situation is similar for node PF when issuing all the vectors resulting from the IDA algorithm. In the second experiment, the topology shown in Fig. 4 is evaluated. In this case IDA and network coding are combined through the implementation of two butterfly schemes. Each butterfly applies network coding for the data streams coming from node PF. The nodes R work as peers and transmit the dispersal in a collaborative way. The network coding scheme used was the traditional network coding scheme, which is based on the use of arithmetic operations such as the binary XOR operation.

We measured the execution times for both experiments using two methods. The first method counts the time required by the processor, while the second method counts the real time of the simulator application, giving an expectation of the possible waiting time scenario for a user. In this way, the receiving nodes, which are the first nodes to be executed, accumulate the logs of the reception times. Results are shown in Figs. 5 and 6. We can see in Fig. 5 (IDA over TCP) the time costs for the execution of the simulator in simple transmissions of the scattered vectors. For a file of 1MB, we obtain a time of 0.632844 s for the processor, and a total time of 12.77619012 s (real time), which is the time it took for the simulator program to recover the complete source vector between each receiver. Figure 6 shows the results obtained from experiments using IDA with network coding. Here, we can observe that the transmission of a 1MB vector requires a processor time of 0.616914 s, while the total real time for the execution and termination of the simulator is 6.31214858 s.

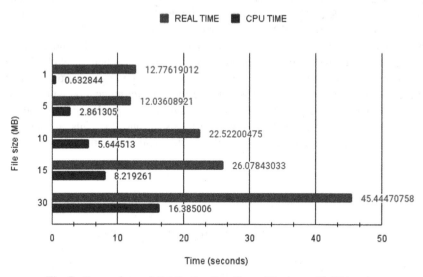

Fig. 5. Comparison of distribution time for architecture with IDA only.

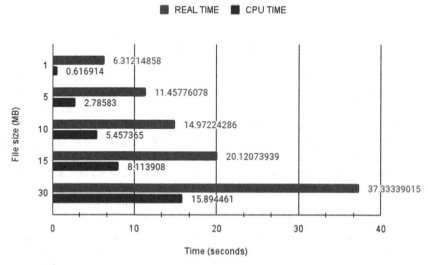

Fig. 6. Comparison of distribution time for architecture with IDA and network coding.

The used methods show that the CPU times could increase with the use of the network coding, because the intermediate nodes require more processing to perform the necessary operations of the schema. This could mean that the proposed architecture may generate a higher cost over time. However, the figures of real seconds, allow to visualize an expectation of the real time for the users (nodes R in Fig. 4) of the architecture. On the other hand, delivery time variations can be observed for different sizes of the source vector. We can also observe that for small vectors (e.g.: 1 MB and 10 MB) it might be convenient to use the proposed architecture. We are evaluating the performance of this architecture using larger vectors.

6   Conclusions

Content delivery plays an important role in the current communication networks. Because these services demand efficient distribution schemes. Network coding and the information dispersal algorithm (IDA) are techniques used to mainly improve the throughput of the communication networks and fault tolerance in the storage systems, respectively. Several applications using both techniques can be found in literature, but separately. In this work, we propose a distributed architecture which combines network coding with IDA to evaluate the impact of this strategy. Our work is in progress, and the preliminary results show that network coding combined with IDA can reduce the delivery time for files of small size. Our implementation has been done using TCP. Therefore, some specific characteristics of TCP such as retransmission of loss packets is very important. Requesting nodes working as peers play an important role because it allows these to work as relay nodes and not as simple leaves of a tree.

As future work we plan continue our experiments evaluating larger files to observe the behavior of our architecture under these scenarios. In addition, we are working in an implementation of our architecture using UDP in order to compare its performance with our implementation done in TCP. Data privacy can also be implemented in our architecture by using encryption techniques based on the AES algorithm.

References

1. Rabin, M.O.: Efficient dispersal of information for security, load balancing, and fault tolerance. J. ACM **36**, 335–3348 (1989)
2. Ahlswede, R., Cai, N., Li, S.-Y., Yeung, R.W.: Network information flow. IEEE Trans. Inf. Theory **46**, 1204–1216 (2000)
3. Chou, P., Wu, Y., Jain, K.: Practical network coding. In: 51st Allerton Conference on Communication, Control and Computation, Monticello, IL, USA (2003)
4. Gkantsidis, C., Rodriguez, P.R.: Network coding for large scale content distribution. In: IEEE INFOCOM 2005, Miami, FL, USA, pp. 2235–2245 (2005)
5. Sundararajan, J.K., Shah, D., Medard, M., Mitzenmache, M., Barros, J.: Network coding meets TCP. In: IEEE INFOCOMM 2009, Rio de Janeiro, Brazil, pp. 280–288 (2009)
6. Androutsellis-Theotokis, S., Spinellis, D.: A survey of peer-to-peer content distribution technologies. ACM Comput. Surv. **36**(4), 335–371 (2004)
7. Milojicic, D.S., et al.: Peer-to-peer computing. Technical report HPL-2002-57R1, HP Labs, Palo Alto (2002)
8. Ripeanu, M., Foster, I., Iamnitchi, A., Rogers, A.: In search for simplicity: a self organizing multi-source multicast overlay. In: 1st IEEE International Conference (SASO 2007), Boston, MA, USA, pp. 371–374 (2007)

9. Santifaller, M.: TCP/IP and NFS Internetworking in UNIX Environment. Addison-Wesley, Boston (1981)

10. Weatherspoon, H., Kubiatowicz, J.D.: Erasure coding vs. replication: a quantitative comparison. In: Druschel, P., Kaashoek, F., Rowstron, A. (eds.) IPTPS 2002. LNCS, vol. 2429, pp. 328–337. Springer, Heidelberg (2002). https://doi.org/10.1007/3-540-45748-8_31

11. Bhagwan, R., Moore, D., Savage, S., Voelker, G.M.: Replication strategies for highly available peer-to-peer storage. In: Schiper, A., Shvartsman, A.A., Weatherspoon, H., Zhao, B.Y. (eds.) Future Directions in Distributed Computing. LNCS, vol. 2584, pp. 153–158. Springer, Heidelberg (2003). https://doi.org/10.1007/3-540-37795-6_28

12. Acedanski, S., Deb, S., Médard, M., Koetter, R.: How good is random linear coding based distributed networked storage? In: 1st Workshop on Network Coding, Theory, and Applications (NetCod) (2005)

13. Rodrigues, R., Liskov, B.: High availability in DHTs: erasure coding vs. replication. In: Castro, M., van Renesse, R. (eds.) IPTPS 2005. LNCS, vol. 3640, pp. 226–239. Springer, Heidelberg (2005). https://doi.org/10.1007/11558989_21

14. Blake, C., Rodrigues, R.: High availability, scalable storage, dynamic peer networks: pick two. In: HOTOS 2003: Proceedings of the 9th conference on Hot Topics in Operating Systems, pp. 1–6 (2003)

15. Dimakis, A.: Network coding for distributed storage systems. In: INFOCOM 2007. 26th IEEE International Conference on Computer Communications, pp. 2000–2008 (2007)

16. Derek, L., Ho, T., Cathey, R.: Optimal content delivery with network coding. In: 43rd Annual Conference on Information Sciences and Systems, CISS 2009, pp. 414–419 (2009)

17. Kwon, M., Kwon, J., Park, B., Park, H.: An architecture of IPTV networks based on network coding. In: International Conference on Ubiquitous Future Networks ICUFN, pp. 462–464 (2017)

18. López Fuentes, F.A., Mendoza Almanza, J., Marcelin-Jiménez, R., Velázquez-Méndez, B.: Efficient content distribution and storage P2P system based on information dispersal. In: 6th International Conference on Control, Decision and Information Technologies (CoDIT) (2019)

19. Mendoza-Almanza, J., López-Fuentes, F.A.: Optimal network coding based on machine learning methods for collaborative networks. In: 6th International Conference on Control, Decision and Information Technologies (CoDIT) (2019)

20. Noura, H.N., Melki, R., Chehab, A., Hernandez-Fernandez, J.: Efficient and robust data availability solution for hybrid PLC/RF systems. In: Computer Networks (2021)

21. Omote, K., Tran, P.T.: ND-POR: a POR based on network coding and dispersal coding. IEICE Trans. Syst. **E98-D**(8), 1465–1476 (2015)

Sentiment Analysis Model on Twitter About Video Streaming Platforms in Mexico

Rosalia Andrade-Gonzalez[1] and Roman Rodriguez-Aguilar[2]([✉]) [iD]

[1] Facultad de Ingenieria, Universidad Anahuac Mexico, Mexico City, Mexico
[2] Facultad de Ciencias Económicas y Empresariales, Universidad Panamericana, Augusto Rodin 498, 03920 Mexico City, Mexico
rrodrigueza@up.edu.mx

Abstract. This work addresses the analysis of the content of the comments on Twitter in the period from December 2020 to February 2021 on the video streaming platforms in Mexico: Netflix, Disney+ and Prime Video. The analysis involves the extraction of comments on Twitter, cleaning the text and the development of a supervised support model for Text Mining for the sentiment classification of tweets in the categories: Positive, Negative or Neutral (spam); as well as the use of resampling techniques to measure the variability of the model's performance and improve the precision of its parameters. The result allows the measurement of user satisfaction levels and the detection of the most dissatisfied and liked aspects of the platforms. Finally, a business intelligence dashboard was developed in Power BI for the interactive visualization of the results under different information filters.

The results show that there is a large percentage of Neutral tweets (spam) that refer mainly to advertising about new releases. Netflix's satisfaction level is the highest compared to the rest of the platforms due to the liking for its original series, variety, and dynamism of launches; on the contrary, the most unpleasant aspect is removing content from your catalog. For its part, Disney+ has satisfaction lower due to the limited variety of its catalog and the expense involved. In the case of Prime Video, lower levels of satisfaction are observed for removing content from its catalog and for paying more than one platform per month. The application of this methodology could benefit in measurement of satisfaction levels, understanding, decision-making and monitoring of new strategies implemented by the platforms.

Keywords: Text mining · Sentiment analysis · Analytical intelligence · Streaming · Satisfaction levels

1 Introduction

Streaming is a technology that allows you to view an audio or video file directly from an Internet page or a mobile application, without completely downloading it to a device. In other words, it is displayed as it is downloaded to a smart TV, computer, tablet, or phone [1].

© ICST Institute for Computer Sciences, Social Informatics and Telecommunications Engineering 2021
Published by Springer Nature Switzerland AG 2021. All Rights Reserved
J. A. Marmolejo-Saucedo et al. (Eds.): COMPSE 2021, LNICST 393, pp. 73–87, 2021.
https://doi.org/10.1007/978-3-030-87495-7_6

The market in Mexico has been led by Netflix since it arrived in the country in 2011 but the launches of new video streaming services continue, with more and more platforms with different business models being added to the market, such as the launch of Disney+ at the end of 2020. Until June 2020, Netflix covered 50% of the users of the video platforms followed by Claro Video and Amazon Prime [2]. However, for September of the same year, Netflix's share fell to 36%, as did Claro Video's share, moving to third position due to the increase in Prime Video's share with 22% of the market. In addition to this, the launch of the new Disney+ platform, at the end of the same year, increases competition.

According to Patrick O'Neill, co-founder of Sherlock Communications "The concern is not about the quality of the programs, but rather with so many options and new competitors preparing to land in Latin America, the ocean of available content could generate 'fatigue of decision 'on users. However, aware of this challenge, the platforms are now looking to improve their recommendation algorithms, all based on big data". The most used video streaming platforms in the Mexican Republic and which will be analyzed in this paper are Netflix and Prime Video as well as the new platform Disney+ due to its recent launch.

Netflix is the platform with the highest price but in variety and quantity, it is the one with the largest offer. Its offer is aimed at all types of public and even with the arrival of new competitors, it continues to be the main platform. Much of its success lies in its commitment to its own content and dynamism in its launches. One of the closest competitors for Netflix is Prime Video, thanks to the large number of people who have already established a relationship with the online sales giant Amazon, and that unlike other platform, it has decided to compete with its rivals offering subscriptions at low prices to attract new customers. The platform provides access to two types of content, the one included in the membership and the one that can be rented or purchased at affordable prices, it also allows you to watch the first episode of selected series for free. In addition, subscribers have access to an Amazon Music account, priority in order delivery from the online store, among others. However, its interface can be a bit more complex and varies in style from device to device. While this platform has 4,295 titles, these tend to be older and while it has been investing in its own original content and in the long term it is probably the right strategy, it is currently not enough to displace Netflix [3].

On the other hand, Disney+ is a platform focused on family entertainment, aimed mainly at children's audiences with limited adult content, which is one of the most common criticisms that the platform receives in addition to the fact that the pace of its launches is slow and has the fewest titles in its catalog. As of September 2019, Netflix had 6,783,000 active accounts and Prime Video served 465,000 customers [4].

Twitter is a platform that has become a news and trends portal with 240 million users worldwide. It is a social network focused purely on informing and in many countries, it is used mainly to be informed and aware of the latest news or official announcements made by different government entities, political figures, and opinion leaders in the world. In general, the age range that dominates this social network ranges from 18 years to 34 years, which covers 53% [5]. In 2020, Twitter was the fifth most used platform in Mexico with 57% participation, the country ranks number 10 in the top reach of Twitter worldwide and is one of the 5 countries that exceeds the average reach with 10% in January 2020 [6].

The number of monthly active users of Twitter exceeded 9.5 million, which represents an increase of almost 24% compared to that registered in the same month of the previous year. It has also been identified that most of the user's access through devices with Android systems with 6.7 million users (70%), although the proportion of users of iOS systems has increased since April 2020 [7]. Twitter began using the hashtag as a method of indexing keywords that would help facilitate good search results to see the top posts surrounding a specific hashtag and participate in the latest trends. The concept was first used in 2007 and since then most social networks have taken advantage of hashtags for the same purpose.

Hashtags that spread quickly and are used by a wide variety of users become trending. This means that a keyword is popular and is being used by many people online. They are an effective way to increase interactions and build a brand when they are using promotional material, when announcing new launches or to generate interest towards the business, they are also helpful in finding a target audience [8]. One way to connect with other users on Twitter is to use mentions, these are dealt with by putting the at symbol (@) in front of the name of a particular user within the content of the tweet. With mentions, users can quote people related to their publication and attract their attention [9].

Text Mining is an interdisciplinary field that involves the modeling of unstructured data to extract useful and high-quality information or knowledge from text by creating patterns and trends taking advantage of numerous statistical techniques of machine learning and computational linguistics [10].

Sentiment analysis refers to the different methods of computational linguistics that help identify and extract subjective information from existing content in the digital world (social networks, forums, websites, etc.). It extracts a tangible and direct value, such as determining whether a text taken from the Internet contains positive or negative connotations [11].

In studies about sentiment analysis, Machine Learning algorithms such as Naive Bayes, Linear Regression, Support Vector Machines and Neural Networks are commonly used. Most of the research and dictionaries are developed in the English language, so there is a need to develop ad hoc tools for the case of each language, also considering the idioms of each region and the expressions used in social networks.

There are studies on the analysis of sentiment of comments on Twitter in the Spanish language applied to other topics, such as Customer Voice Analysis [12]. However, there is no research on sentiment analysis in Twitter comments about streaming platforms in Mexico.

In recent years, the number of platforms that offer new video streaming services in Mexico with different business models has increased due to the profitability of this technology and the great acceptance by users as it is a practical and economical option. Increased competition implies a new challenge for platforms with a significant positioning in the current market such as Netflix or Prime Video, and on the other hand it implies a significant challenge for new platforms seeking to position themselves in the market such as Disney+. For this, it is important to consider the perception of current and potential clients of the platforms through social networks and measure satisfaction levels by identifying the aspects of greatest liking, dissatisfaction or even failures of each platform in the face of the demanding demand for content by users and the strategies of their competitors. The objective of this work is to measure satisfaction levels through customer sentiment towards the main video streaming platforms, using a sentiment classification model for posts on Twitter in Mexico. The work is structured as follows, in section two the materials and methods are described, section three presents the main results and finally the conclusions and references.

2 Materials and Methods

2.1 Description of the Data

For the compilation of the information and construction of the database, Twitter Archiver was used, which is a tool that searches for tweets by means of a keyword or hashtag, saving the matching tweets in a Google spreadsheet automatically. So that every hour it searches and extracts all the new tweets accumulating them in the spreadsheet [13]. The tool was used to compile the databases of the tweets from each of the platforms separately in the period from December 2020 to February 2021. Later they were downloaded and by programming in R, they were consolidated into a single database with 436,110 records in total.

In general, texts can be grammatically complex and in the case of comments on social networks, such as those on Twitter, it can find many empty words, punctuation marks, spelling mistakes and words with a lot or little frequency that do not contribute to decipher the actual content of the comment. For this reason, any data analysis process begins with a preliminary step that includes pre-processing, cleaning, and exploratory analysis. To get the meaning of a text, a measure is needed so quantitative data is first extracted by processing the text with various transformation methods. Although there is no single methodology to perform text preprocessing and cleaning, each technique seeks to discard unnecessary information and there are various methods, packages, APIs, and software that can transform text into quantitative data. In the case of R, there are packages that clean the text mainly in English, so in this work we will develop a process of cleaning the text itself, focused on the data with which it is working and with the flexibility of be able to adapt it to other texts.

For the purposes of this work, a V-Corpus will be used, with the purpose of converting each of the tweets into a different document and that the entire collection is temporarily stored in memory. Once the separation has been carried out in different documents, the Tokenization method will be used, which is the process of separating sequence of characters or a defined document unit, into phrases, words, symbols, or other useful elements called tokens. For the quantitative analysis of the text, they are considered as a collection of words or bag of words and the key words, frequencies of occurrences and the importance of each word in the text are extracted.

The next step is to put together and assume that all tweets are a collection of unique words (bag of words) where frequency and order are irrelevant. It will seek to standardize all words by converting them to lowercase and removing accents, punctuation, special characters, and stop-words. On the other hand, the grammar in any language allows the use of derivationally related words with similar meanings, which are nothing more than a different form of the same word. Therefore, to reduce the inflectional forms and the derived words to the common or infinitive base form a stemming was applied. To find the similarity between words, it is necessary to evaluate how similar they are through distance measure. One way to find the similarity between two words is through "edit distance", which refers to the number of operations required to transform a string of characters, in this case one word, into another, such as the Levenshtein distance. Once the words have been reduced to their inflectional form, another way to unify the words is through the n-grams. An n-gram is a group of n words that are written together frequently.

The initial database consists of 436,110 records of tweets in Spanish language on video streaming platforms: Netflix, Prime Video and Disney+, in the period from December 20, 2020, to February 27, 2021. It has 21 fields provided by the Twitter Archiver tool plus 4 variables calculated from these (Table 1).

Table 1. Description of variables

Name	Description
Date	Tweet publication date
Screen Name	Name of the user who posted the tweet
Full Name	Full name of the user who posted the tweet
Tweet Text	Tweet text
Tweet ID	Tweet id
Link(s)	Link related to the tweet
Media	Link to the image contained in the tweet
Location	Location of the user who posted the tweet
Retweets	Number of retweets from other users to the published tweet
Favorites	Number of users who added the published tweet to their favorites
App	Application used to post the tweet
Followers	Number of user followers
Follows	Number of users the user follows
Listed	Number of user lists
Verified	Indicates if the account is verified or not
User Since	User creation date on Twitter
Location	User's location
Bio	Biography of the user in his profile
Website	User website
Time zone	Time zone
Profile Image	User profile photo link

(*continued*)

Table 1. (*continued*)

Name	Description
Years of antiquity	Years of seniority of the user on Twitter
Platform	Streaming platform mentioned in the tweet
Frequency	Number of times the same tweet was published in the analysis period
Unique users' frequency	Number of different users who published the same tweet in the analysis period

2.2 Structure of the Proposed Model

The structure of the process for measuring customer satisfaction levels on video stream-ing platforms in Mexico is based on the results of the sentiment prediction model of posts on Twitter, consists of collecting and downloading tweets about the platforms in a certain period with Google's Tweet Archiver tool. The databases will be read and consolidated with the R program, which will also load all the dictionaries required for cleaning text and creating predictor variables. The R program will carry out the text cleaning process, the creation of the variables required for the model and will apply the model to predict the sentiment of the tweets. The construction of the sentiment model started from the manual classification of each twit according to the content in three levels: positive, neg-ative, and neutral sentiment. To select the sentiment classification model to be used, a comparison was made of a set of generally accepted methodologies in machine learning:

- Support vector machines
- K-nearest neighbors
- Decision trees
- Neural networks
- Boosting
- Random forest

The base with the variables provided by the Tweet Archiver tool, those created for the model and the sentiment prediction, will be read by the Power BI tool that generates an interactive visualization board in which the results can be visualized by performing different information filters that will allow to monitor the results over time (Fig. 1).

It is important to highlight that for the definition of the dictionaries, custom dictio-naries based on the Spanish language were used. The base with the variables provided by the Tweet Archiver tool, those created for the model and the sentiment prediction, will be read by the Power BI tool that generates an interactive visualization board in which the results can be visualized by performing different information filters (Fig. 1).

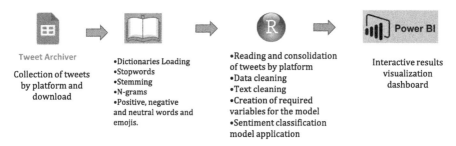

Tweet Archiver

Collection of tweets
by platform and
download

•Dictionaries Loading
•Stopwords
•Stemming
•N-grams
•Positive, negative
and neutral words and
emojis.

•Reading and consolidation
of tweets by platform
•Data cleaning
•Text cleaning
•Creation of required
variables for the model
•Sentiment classification
model application

Power BI

Interactive results
visualization
dashboard

Fig. 1. Proposed model.

3   Results

3.1   Text Cleaning and Debugging

After the exploratory analysis for a better understanding of the information and cleaning of both variables and records, there is a final base with 35,173 records to continue cleaning the text of the tweets. The text cleaning process consisted of the extraction of hashtags and mentions, text standardization, emoji translation, definition of Stop words, Stemming, definition of Bigrams and Trigrams and selection by criteria of Frequency of words. Later all the text cleaning actions, only 17% of the initial number of unique words (15, 068) is preserved, which are only the most relevant words that will help to build the sentiment model. To identify if users mention more than one platform in the same tweet to make a comparison or promotion between them, 3 indicator variables were created, one for each platform, which indicate whether the pattern sought corresponding to each platform. It is found within the text of the tweet using regular expressions. With this, it was possible to identify that 97% only refer to 1 platform while 3% mention 2 to 3 platforms in the same tweet. A new variable was created with the percentage of characters removed per tweet with the text cleanup calculated as Eq. 1.

$$\left(\frac{\text{Length of original tweet} - \text{Length of clean tweet}}{\text{Length of original tweet}} \right) * 100 \tag{1}$$

That indicates the percentage of irrelevant and discarded words from the original tweet, which can be an important predictor of sentiment. When analyzing the distribution of the variable, it was found that on average 51% of the characters of each tweet were eliminated with the cleaning actions (Fig. 2).

To analyze the content of the tweets, word clouds were created for each platform and variable: Tweet text, Hashtags, Mentions (@) and Translation of emojis to text. The most common terms in the tweets about Netflix are about its series, documentaries, and new releases; while in publications about Disney+ and Prime video, the terms related to its catalog of films and premieres are more frequent (Fig. 3).

In the case of emojis, it is a variable that can provide relevant information for the sentiment classification, so they were transformed into text and will be used as an additional explanatory variable for the sentiment classification model.

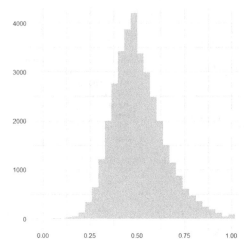

Fig. 2. Distribution of the percentage of character removal by cleaning.

3.2 Sentiment Classification Model

A correlation analysis was performed between the base variables with the 35,173 records, to identify the correlated variables, that is, those that contain the same information to select independent variables for model training. A manual classification of sentiment was performed: Positive, Negative or Neutral, of a random sample of 30% (10,487 tweets) of the total base tweets with the aim of training the model. With the results of the classification, a preliminary analysis was carried out where it was found that 57% of the tweets have Neutral sentiment (spam), 22% Negative and 20% Positive.

By platform, Netflix has the same proportion of Positive and Negative tweets (21%) while Disney+ has a higher proportion of Negative comments (24%) compared to Positive ones (19%) and Prime Video has a higher proportion of Neutral tweets (spam) (62%) and an almost equal proportion between Positive and Negative tweets (18–19%) (Fig. 4).

Word clouds were made by platform and sentiment to identify the main words of each one. As a result of the word clouds, it is observed that the main reasons for Negative tweets about Netflix are due to removing movies/series from its catalog, not having them, being bad or due to the payment of the platform without seeing its content or the expense that caused by being the most expensive. On the other hand, Positive tweets refer to the fact that they like the content and recommend it for being good options, they also express appreciation for documentaries, seasons, and award nominations. For its part, Disney+ has a greater variety of Negative words, since users express various reasons, such as canceling the subscription for not wanting to pay for a new platform in addition to the existing offer, limited/bad catalog, or dissatisfaction with the fall of the platform due to saturation due to the weekly premiere (such as new chapter of "WandaVision"). However, the Positive comments refer to the fact that the platform has the best/favorite films of the users that provoke positive emotions and childhood memories or show liking for new film success stories (such as "The Mandalorian"). In the case of the Prime Video platform, users publish Negative tweets mainly because of movies they remove from the

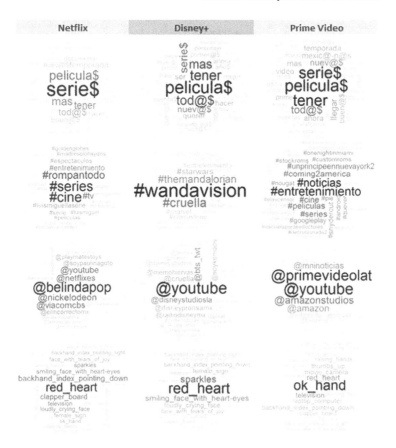

Fig. 3. Word clouds by platform and text of the tweet, hashtags, mentions and emojis.

catalog or because they are paying for the platform without occupying it, having bad content or because of the ads that are shown. On the other hand, Positive tweets refer to the fact that the platform contains good options for movies that users consider to be the best (Fig. 5).

From the sample of the base with the manual classification of the sentiment of the tweets, the main words that influence the classification of the sentiment were identified as a "catalog" of words by sentiment. As a criterion for the selection of the main words of each feeling, those with the highest frequency were considered from a certain percentile. Similarly, a "catalog" of Positive, Negative and Neutral (spam) emojis was established based on the frequency of the emojis to assign them in a sentiment category.

Finally, there is a base with 23 variables for calculating the optimal percentile to establish the "catalogs" of feeling words with which to obtain greater effectiveness in training the sentiment classification model. To determine the optimal percentile to establish the "catalog" of each sentiment, a cross-validation process was carried out with all possible combinations of percentiles in multiples of 25%, in which the classification models were tested: Support Vector Machines, KNN, Naive Bayes, Decision Tree and

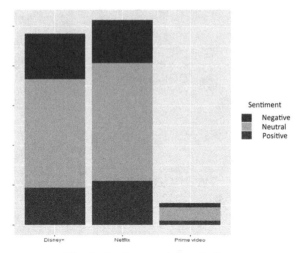

Fig. 4. Sentiment ratio per platform

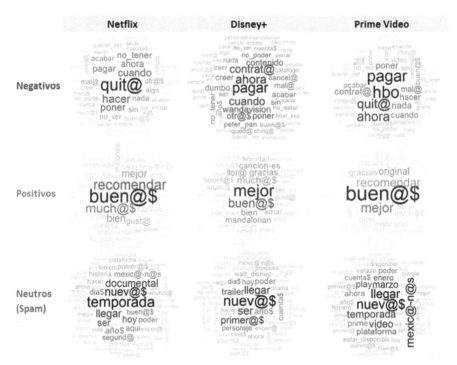

Fig. 5. Word clouds by platform and sentiment of the base sample with manual classification for model training.

Neural Network, with the default parameters and considering a base segmentation of 50% for training and 50% for validation. To measure the effectiveness of the models in each combination, the misclassification rate was calculated to choose the combination of percentiles per sentiment that minimizes the error in most of the models and in turn maximizes the percentiles so that the "catalogs" contain the fewest possible words.

With the result of the cross-validation, the optimal 50th percentile was determined for each sentiment and the three "catalogs" were formed, consisting of 1,525 Positive words, 1,035 Negative words and 3,548 Neutral words. The definition of the optimal percentile to generate the "catalogs" of words by sentiment and form the table with the final variables of best effectiveness in all the models with the default parameters, the optimization of the parameters will be sought, minimizing the misclassification rate by validation with 50% of the base as training and 50% for validation.

The misclassification rate of each model was calculated under different seeds and percentages of the size of the training and validation base to measure the variability of each model under different scenarios and to determine the average effectiveness. As a result, the models with the lowest average rate were Boosting (18.0%) and Polynomial Support Vector Machine (18.4%). However, when applying the model to the validation data with the different percentages of sample and seeds, it was obtained that the best model is the Linear Support Vector Machine with an average misclassification rate of 22.7% (Table 2).

Table 2. Misclassified rate (%) of validation by percentage of sample and seed

%		Validation Sample							
		SVM Lineal	SVM Radial	SVM Polynomial	KNN	NN	Pruned tree	Random Forest	Boosting
50%	Seed 1	23.0	24.3	26.3	27.0	23.6	28.6	22.8	24.0
	Seed 2	23.0	24.3	26.3	27.1	24.3	28.6	23.2	23.4
	Seed 3	23.0	24.3	26.3	26.9	24.3	28.6	23.1	23.6
40%	Seed 1	23.6	24.4	26.6	27.7	23.3	28.1	23.5	23.9
	Seed 2	23.6	24.4	26.6	27.4	23.9	28.1	23.5	23.6
	Seed 3	23.6	24.4	26.6	27.5	23.8	28.1	23.7	23.9
30%	Seed 1	22.8	23.0	25.2	26.2	22.8	27.3	23.4	24.6
	Seed 2	22.8	23.0	25.2	26.2	22.7	27.3	23.2	24.0
	Seed 3	22.8	23.0	25.2	26.1	22.8	27.3	23.5	24.4
20%	Seed 1	22.3	23.4	24.4	25.8	22.8	27.3	23.1	21.7
	Seed 2	22.3	23.4	24.4	25.8	22.0	27.3	23.4	22.4
	Seed 3	22.3	23.4	24.4	25.7	22.6	27.3	23.5	22.5
10%	Seed 1	22.0	23.0	25.1	28.7	23.5	26.5	23.4	22.5
	Seed 2	22.0	23.0	25.1	28.6	23.1	26.5	23.8	22.6
	Seed 3	22.0	23.0	25.1	28.6	23.0	26.5	23.5	23.0
Average		22.7	23.6	25.5	27.0	23.2	27.6	23.4	23.2

The most effective model to model the sentiment of tweets is the Linear Support Vector Machine with a cost of 0.01, which has a 77% average effectiveness, which implies a misclassification error of 23%. When applying the model to the total base of tweets, it was determined that in general, 65% of tweets are Neutral (spam), 19% have Negative sentiment and 16% Positive. Analyzing the proportion by platform it was found that there is a greater proportion of Negative comments compared to Positive in the case of Disney+ with 20% and 15%, respectively. On the other hand, Netflix shows a similar proportion of Positive and Negative (17% and 18%). Compared to the other platforms, Prime video has a higher proportion of Neutral tweets (spam) with 71% and presents a higher percentage of Negative tweets (17%) compared to Positive ones (12%).

3.3 Interactive Display Board

An interactive visualization dashboard was developed with the Microsoft business analysis tool Power BI, to facilitate the visualization of the results, perform ad hoc filters and monitor the content of tweets on video streaming platforms through weather. The board consists in two sections. General section contains the total number of tweets and graphs with the proportion of tweets by platform, sentiment, and APP as well as the trend of the number of daily tweets by platform and a map of the Republic of Mexico that shows the number of tweets by state. The percentage of users with the website and the percentage of tweets with links and images or photos in the publication is displayed. It also shows the average number of tweets, antiquity, followers, follows and length of biography per user and the table with the details of each user (Fig. 6).

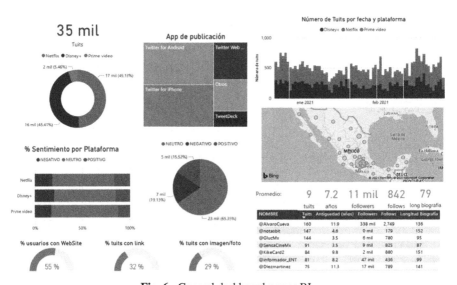

Fig. 6. General dashboard power BI.

The word cloud section contains the word clouds of tweets, hashtags, at and emojis with the option to filter them by platform and sentiment. It will also display the average number of characters of the tweets originally and the percentage that is removed after the cleaning process; as well as the percentages of tweets that contain at least one hashtag, mentions and emojis (Fig. 7).

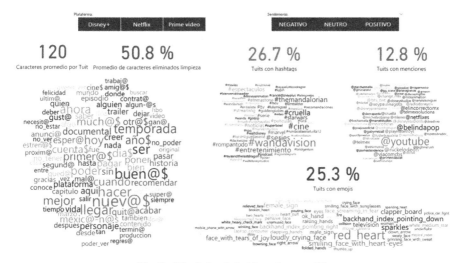

Fig. 7. Word cloud dashboard power BI.

4   Conclusions

The Text Mining application focused on the analysis of sentiment in social networks on streaming video platforms is a new proposal that helps to extract useful and easy to understand information about what users are expressing in relation to the service and content offered with the objective to help decision-making by analyzing the impact of increasing competition in the sector. In the development process, text cleaning is the most complex part due to the absence of catalogs in different languages or idioms used by different regions and in social networks, which implies developing an ad hoc solution with the analyzed context. In the present work, Spanish-language dictionaries applicable to texts related to video streaming platforms were developed because of a process designed for the pre-processing and cleaning of texts for periodic updating or applicable to other types of texts in the Spanish language.

Netflix has led the video streaming platform market in Mexico for being the first since its arrival in 2011 with the largest number of users, variety, and original content; However, with the increase in competition, its percentage of market share has decreased, and it has diversified among the rest of the platforms in recent years; one of the main reasons is because the platform has the highest price in the market. Its main competition is Prime Video, a platform that has penetrated the market due to its relationship with Amazon and its attractive price; However, the platform does not register a significant number of tweets for sentiment analysis and most of the posts are advertising. On the other hand, the launch of the new Disney+ platform has registered a high volume of publications like Netflix and its main attraction is its children's content and the launch of new film success stories.

To clean the text of the tweets, dictionaries of stop words, stemming, n-grams were elaborated, and various techniques were applied to reduce the number of irrelevant words in the tweets for the sentiment analysis, keeping on average only half of the words in every tweet. A manual classification of a sample of tweets was also carried out in each sentiment to develop catalogs of words and emojis per sentiment for the training of the model based on a cross-validation process that minimized the classification error in all the models.

It was determined that the best sentiment classification model is a Linear Support Vector Machine with an average classification error of 22.7%. Applying the model, 65% of the tweets have Neutral sentiment (spam) and most are published by official accounts of users with a greater number of publications, followers, character length in their biography, hashtags within the tweets and a greater proportion of words removed with the text cleaning process.

Netflix's satisfaction levels are the best as it has an equitable ratio between Positive and Negative tweets, this due to its liking for its content, mainly from original series; on the contrary, the aspect of greatest discontent is removing content from its catalog. For its part, the entry of Disney+ to the Mexican market was well received; However, the level of satisfaction is lower due to the limited variety of its catalog and the expense involved, considering that users already have some other platform. In the case of Prime Video, lower levels of satisfaction are observed for removing content from its catalog and for paying more than one platform per month. All the results can be observed interactively through a visualization board (dashboard) developed in Power BI in which ad hoc filters, analysis can be carried out, and the content of tweets on video streaming platforms can be tracked through time.

References

1. Selectra. Streaming: qué es, cómo funciona, precios y periodo de prueba 2020 (2020). Recuperado de https://selectra.mx/streaming#que-es-el-streaming
2. EL CEO. Netflix perderá concentración de mercado en México por más plataformas de streaming (2020). Recuperado de https://elceo.com/tecnologia/netflix-perdera-concentracion-de-mercado-en-mexico-por-mas-plataformas-de-streaming/
3. Sin embargo, Dávila, A.L.: El streaming convierte 2020 en su mejor año en la historia, y prepara grandes sorpresas para 2021 (2020). Recuperado de https://www.sinembargo.mx/24-12-2020/3913008
4. El Universal, Lucas, N.: México cerró el 2019 con más de 10 millones de cuentas OTT pagadas (2019). Recuperado de https://www.eleconomista.com.mx/empresas/Mexico-cerro-el-2019-con-mas-de-10-millones-de-cuentas-OTT-pagadas-20200122-0052.html
5. Yi MiN Shum Xie. Resumen de Twitter 2020 (2020). Recuperado de https://yiminshum.com/twitter-digital-2020/
6. Statista. Redes sociales con el mayor porcentaje de usuarios en México en 2020 (2020). Recuperado de https://es.statista.com/estadisticas/1035031/mexico-porcentaje-de-usuarios-por-red-social/

7. Statista. Número de usuarios activos mensuales (MAU) de Twitter en México de enero de 2019 a agosto de 2020, por sistema operative (2020). Recuperado de https://es.statista.com/estadisticas/1172236/numero-de-usuarios-activos-mensuales-twitter-mexico-sistema-operativo/

8. Hootsuite, Adame, A.: Cómo utilizar hashtags: una guía rápida y sencilla para cada red social (2019). Recuperado de https://blog.hootsuite.com/es/hashtags-la-guia-completa/

9. Postcron, Skaf, E.: Cómo usar Twitter: 15 tips indispensables (2019). Recuperado de https://postcron.com/es/blog/como-usar-twitter/#:~:text=Para%20esto%2C%20basta%20con%20anteponer,asegurarte%20de%20que%20la%20vean

10. Kumar, A., Paul, A.: Mastering Text Mining with R. Packt Publishing, Birmingham (2016)

11. ITELLIGENT. Análisis de sentimiento, ¿qué es, cómo funciona y para qué sirve? (2017). Recuperado de https://itelligent.es/es/analisis-de-sentimiento/

12. Gonzalez, R.A., Rodriguez-Aguilar, R., Marmolejo-Saucedo, J.A.: Text mining and statistical learning for the analysis of the voice of the customer. In: Hemanth, D.J., Kose, U. (eds.) ICAIAME 2019. LNDECT, vol. 43, pp. 191–199. Springer, Cham (2020). https://doi.org/10.1007/978-3-030-36178-5_16

13. Digital inspiration. Save Tuits in Google Sheets (2015). Recuperado de https://digitalinspiration.com/product/twitter-archiver

14. Hastie, T., Tibshirani, R., Friedman, J.: The Elements of Statistical Learning. Springer, Stanford (2008)

15. del Carmen, V.P.M., Covarrubias, C.C.: Identificación del color en video en tiempo real solución estadística a un problema computacional. Tesis Universidad Anáhuac México, México (2017)

16. Decision Tree Modeling. Course Notes. Ed. SAS Education ISBN 978-1-59994-280-3

17. Neural Network Modeling. Course Notes, Ed. SAS Education ISBN 978-1-59047-771-7

An Asset Index Proposal for Households in Mexico Applying the Mixed Principal Components Analysis Methodology

Lorena DelaTorre-Díaz$^{(\boxtimes)}$ and Román Rodriguez-Aguilar

Facultad de Ciencias Económicas y Empresariales, Universidad Panamericana, Augusto Rodin 498, 03920 Mexico City, Mexico
lotorre@up.edu.mx

Abstract. The development of assets indices has grown as an alternative to measure wealth from different generations in the evaluation of social mobility. A proposal of the development of an asset index is presented using the GSVD-based mixed principal components analysis (PCAMix package in R). The contribution rests in the combination of both numerical and categorical data and the integration of the simultaneous effect of these variables in the index. It was used in profiling the Mexican households according to the information from the 2018 National Household Income and Expenditure and the determination of the Gini coefficient to evaluate the inequality of distribution at the state level. Results show a high level of disparity in the distribution of assets with only 0.01% of the households possessing 40% or more of the assets included in the index, being the southern region where greatest challenges for ascending social mobility.

Keywords: Asset index · Mixed principal components · Social mobility · Mexico

1 Introduction

Social mobility refers to the changes experienced by individuals in their socioeconomic condition, reflected in a variation in their relative position according to an educational, employment or income indicator [1, 2]. Its analysis makes it possible to determine whether aspects such as effort and talent determine the achievement of objectives and the change in their living conditions, regardless of the individual's physical and personal characteristics or the socioeconomic position of their parents [3].

A society that favors social mobility allows individuals to improve their living status on their own merits and are not predetermined by their conditions of origin. Social mobility is therefore one of the aspects of the study of inequality of opportunities in a society.

The World Economic Forum [4] recently developed the Global Social Mobility Index (GSMI) that offers a tool to identify areas for improvement in this indicator, evaluating ten pillars: health, education access, education quality and equity, lifelong

© ICST Institute for Computer Sciences, Social Informatics and Telecommunications Engineering 2021
Published by Springer Nature Switzerland AG 2021. All Rights Reserved
J. A. Marmolejo-Saucedo et al. (Eds.): COMPSE 2021, LNICST 393, pp. 88–106, 2021.
https://doi.org/10.1007/978-3-030-87495-7_7

learning, social protection, technology access, work opportunities, fair wages, working conditions, efficient and inclusive institutions. In the first edition, 82 countries were compared with 51 indicators. In the results report, it is estimated that an increase of 10 points in the index could translate into an additional growth in GDP of 4.41% by 2030. Hence the importance for countries to identify and invest in the right mix of factors determinants of social mobility. Mexico was ranked 58th out of the 82 countries evaluated, with the Nordic economies showing the best levels of social mobility and therefore greater equality of opportunities for their population.

Countries with greater inequality experience less mobility between generations, as a greater fraction of the economic advantages and disadvantages are passed from parents to children. This relationship is represented by the so-called Great Gatsby Curve, which is constructed using income inequality measured by the Gini Coefficient on the horizontal axis, and a measure of intergenerational economic mobility on the vertical axis [5].

This curve highlights that inequality of opportunities is the missing link between income inequality and social mobility: if greater inequality makes intergenerational mobility more difficult, it is due to greater inequality in the distribution of economic growth opportunities for the new generations.

The measurement of social mobility from an economic perspective has used as the main variable the level of income from wages and salaries or the level of family income that includes other elements such as transfers or financial assets [6]. However, there are studies that propose an alternative estimate based on the wealth of families under the assumption that the accumulation of assets constitutes a better approximation to household wealth [7].

In the economic research literature, different studies can be found that use asset indices as the indicator of economic mobility, in substitution of income level: [6–9] are some examples. These indices can be a valid predictor of the manifestation of poverty, as well as become an approximation of long-term wealth with a lower degree of error than the measurement of expenditures [10].

Particularly in developing countries, the use of asset indices has increased in studies related to poverty and inequality since these indicators present fewer measurement problems or resistance from interviewees to provide the information. Additionally, when comparing asset possessions, it is possible to establish differences in living conditions between households in the same country, between countries or even in periods over time [10, 11]. Most countries periodically prepare national representation surveys that provide this type of data, which favors the creation of these indices and their use in intergenerational analysis.

In Mexico, studies that have developed asset indices have used data from the available specialized social mobility surveys (Encuesta de Movilidad Social [EMOVI by its acronym in Spanish]) from 2006, 2011 and 2017. However, the National Institute of Statistics and Geography (Instituto Nacional de Estadística y Geografía [INEGI by its acronym in Spanish]) provides robust information on the profile and living conditions of households in Mexico obtained through the National Household Income and Expenditure Surveys (Encuesta Nacional de Ingreso y Gasto de los Hogares [ENIGH by its acronym in Spanish]) and this information has not been used for the development of assets indices before. This survey includes not only dichotomous variables, but categorical multi-level variables, as well as qualitative variables derived from a broader objective of offering an overview of the behavior of household income and expenditure, the sociodemographic characteristics of its members and the household infrastructure characteristics.

Moreover, the calculated indices have used methods focused exclusively on numerical or categorical variables, but no asset index has been developed by combining both.

Derived from the above, the present study aims to develop an asset index representing the households in Mexico with the information from ENIGH 2018. The selection of assets that would be part of the index takes as a reference the pillars conforming the Global Social Mobility Index [4], and the mixed principal components method is applied. Additionally, the asset index will be used to rank households in Mexico and compare it with the Gini Coefficient.

The structure of the study is as follows: in Sect. 2 the framework of social mobility is addressed, including a background on the use of asset indices. Section 3 describes the methodology used in the development of the index and the variables selected for the analysis. Section 4 contains the results of the analysis as well as the conclusions obtained and further analysis possibilities.

2   Social Mobility Framework

Social mobility refers to changes in the socioeconomic condition of individuals, and can be defined in educational, employment or income terms [2]. Sociologists study social mobility as changes in class and job configuration, while economists evaluate mobility in terms of an income vector or some other measure of well-being [12].

Social mobility can also be analyzed in its intragenerational dimension, that is, the mobility that the same individual experiences during his or her life, or intergenerational that refers to the mobility of individuals with respect to their parents [13]. Furthermore, mobility can be absolute when it refers to the rise or fall in an absolute income scale, or relative when the change is measured in relation to the position occupied in the reference period [2].

The absence of upward social mobility in a society gives rise to situations such as the loss of potential talents that remain hidden, decrease in productivity levels, loss of investment opportunities, the hoarding of educational, economic or financial opportunities on the part of the higher socioeconomic classes, waste in the allocation of human resources, and finally a breakdown of the social cohesion when citizens perceive barriers that prevent them from accessing better conditions [14, 15].

2.1   Assets Indices for Measuring Social Mobility

The variable that is traditionally used to estimate social mobility in economic terms is income. This variable can include not only income from wages and salaries but also other factors such as financial assets and public and private transfers [6].

Nonetheless, this methodology is limited by the need to have information on the income of different generations, which is not always available in all countries or regions. Therefore, a growing trend in the literature is the development of asset indices that allow estimating household wealth and, based on them, assessing its mobility. These indices can be considered approximations of permanent household income [6, 7, 9].

Although a combination of human, physical, social and financial assets is required to improve the socioeconomic situation of people, the accumulation of physical assets can generate greater wealth, and become a possible indicator of the capacity of that condition improvement [16].

The models of Filmer-Pritchett [17] and Sahn-Stifel [10] are the most cited. The former developed an index of household assets and characteristics based on the principal component analysis methodology (PCA) to assess the impact of wealth on the educational level of households in Brazil, India and Kenya, and later to assess the relationship between wealth and school enrollment in India [18]. The value of the first principal component is the latent variable that represents the possession of household assets.

On the other hand, in [10] and [19] a factor analysis was used to estimate a single common factor that explains the variances in the possession of a set of assets, and this factor is considered as the metric of economic status or well-being.

Other studies followed the PCA methodology for the elaboration of asset indices that are used to measure social mobility in Mexico. One measures educational, occupational, and economic intergenerational social mobility [7]; another uses an asset index to measure intergenerational social mobility in Mexico between 1950 and 1980 [6].

The information from the 2011 Social Mobility Survey (EMOVI) was used in an study where PCA was used to develop the asset index based on three types of assets: consumer durable goods, household features and financial assets including the possession of a bank account, credit card, vacuum cleaner, toaster, domestic service, telephone, savings account, water heater, washing machine, refrigerator, automobile, inside toilet, stove, electricity service, tubing water, own house and the household crowding index [7].

Similarly, the 2006, 2011 and 2017 EMOVI information was used [6] and created an asset index including the ownership of personal computer, cellular phone, landline phone, internet access, cable TV, shop or business, land or farm, second residence, animals, agricultural equipment, stove, washing machine, refrigerator, inside toilet, electricity, domestic service, savings account, checking account, credit cards and cars. In a previous study, [20] it was also included the parents' and respondents' occupation status.

There are examples of studies using PCA in other regions, such as Bangladesh where a wealth index was used in the evaluation of intergenerational mobility [21], in Colombia [22], or in Pakistan [23].

A variation from the previous studies is where it was decided to use the multiple correspondence analysis (MCA) given that most of the variables included in the index were categoric (mostly binaries) [8]. They included additional variables such as vacation home, apartment for rent and investment in shares.

As noted above, most studies have relied on methodologies focused only on numerical variables. However, there are scarce studies reporting the use of a mixed component analysis method, being an example of the use of a multiple-factor-analysis method that handles a combination of quantitative and qualitative variables a study used in the assessment of poverty alleviation programs in China [24].

It is worth to mention that no studies have been identified using mixed principal components analysis in the evaluation of social mobility.

3 Method

3.1 PCAMix Method

The method used for the construction of the asset index in this study is the mixed principal components analysis applying the generalized singular value decomposition methodology (GSVD), given the different nature of the variables selected. The PCA Mix (also called PCA with metrics) is a generalization of standard PCA using the GSVD to decompose the matrix Z obtained after processing the original information in order to have a particular case of PCA for the numerical variables and MCA for the categorical ones [25, 26].

The Z matrix is the real matrix $Z = [Z_1, Z_2]$ of dimension $n \times p$ where Z_1 is the standard version of the $n \, x \, p$ quantitative matrix and Z_2 is the centered version of the $n \times m$ indicator matrix G of the $n \times p$ qualitative matrix (n being the number of observations and p the number of variables).

The standard PCA aims to reduce the number of dimensions under analysis, maintaining the maximum representation of the original information, and even creating a latent measure that takes the form of an index. PCA analysis is useful when the differences or distances between continuous variables can be captured, however its interpretation is less clear when categorical variables are included.

The alternative method of multiple correspondence analysis is constructed using categorical variables and its purpose is also to reduce dimensionality, using the relative frequencies of each category as a substitute for distances [8].

However, when it is desired to generate a latent variable from a combination of quantitative and categorical variables, a mixed method is used [27], maintaining the same objective of reduction of dimensions. The information provided by surveys such as the national income and expenses surveys include different types of variables, and when many of those variables are considered relevant in the evaluation of the household socioeconomic condition, a methodology that uses mixed date is preferred.

In the construction of an asset index using a mixed methodology, the impact of the variable is not only limited to the possession or not of the asset -as it is in the traditional PCA and MCA methods -, but the amount of money the household spends on it.

PCA Mix splits the original dataset into a numerical matrix and a categorical matrix, and then uses PCA on the quantitative variables and MCA on the categorical variables to obtain a linear combination of the observed variables that accounts for the largest inertia (o variance) [24]. Equation 1 shows the decomposition of the matrix Z.

$$Z = U \Lambda V^T \tag{1}$$

Where:

Z is the real matrix of dimension $n \times p$.
N and M are the diagonal matrixes of the weights of the n rows and p columns.

Λ is the diagonal $r \times r$ matrix $(\sqrt{\lambda 1}, \ldots, \sqrt{\lambda r})$ of the singular values of ZMZ^TN and Z^TNZM, where r denotes the rank of Z.

U is the $n \times r$ matrix of the first r eigenvectors of ZMZ^TN where $U^TNU = I_r$ with I_r the identity matrix of size r

V^T is the $p \times r$ matrix of the first r eigenvectors of Z^TNZM such that $V^TMV = I_r$

After the GSVD method, PCA Mix produces a matrix of dimension $(p_1 + m) \times r$ of the factor coordinates of the p_1 quantitative variables and the m levels of the p_2 categorical variables [28].

The decision of the number of dimensions to maintain is based on the proportion of the total inertia for each dimension.

3.2 Measure of Concentration

The Gini coefficient is a common measure of inequality, evaluating the degree of distribution of income or wealth among individuals or households from a perfectly distributed economy. Its values range from cero (a perfectly equitable distribution) to 1, where a single individual or household concentrates wealth [29] (Eq. 2).

$$G = 1 - \frac{2}{N-1}\left(N - \frac{\sum_{i=1}^{N} ix_i}{\sum_{i=1}^{N} x_i}\right) \tag{2}$$

Where N is the population size and x_i is the variable under evaluation of the *ith* individual or household. Although it is commonly used to evaluate the inequality of the distribution of the income, this coefficient can be used to measure the degree of concentration of any variable. In the present study, the Gini coefficient is calculated using the asset index as the proxy for household wealth.

The Gini coefficient from the *reldist* package in R is used. This model was developed by Handcock as one especial case of the models described in Handcock & Morris [30].

3.3 Segmentation

The clustering method of K-mean is used to segment the Mexican states in groups presenting maximum intra-group homogeneity and inter-group heterogeneity [24]. This clustering technique is a form of unsupervised classification, where there is no external criterion used for the grouping of the cases. On the contrary, the groups are formed after evaluating the intrinsic similarities and dissimilarities among the different cases [31].

The k-means clustering from R was used.

3.4 Data and Variables

The information was taken from the ENIGH carried out in 2018. The size of this national coverage sample was 87,826 households representing 125 million inhabitants from Mexico and the dataset is distributed in 11 tables containing normalized data and an additional table offering a household-level summary. The units of analysis are dwelling, household and the members of the household.

The selection of the variables was based on seven of the ten pillars used by the World Economic Forum's Global Social Mobility Index (GSMI) including a group of qualitative variables representing the ownership of different types of assets and services for each household, and a group of quantitative variables that represent the average monthly expenses (or income) destined by (obtained from) each household to certain income/expense activities.

Additionally, other financial-inclusion variables were included, such as possession of credit card, life insurance policy, mortgage, or similar housing loan, the financial and capital monthly perception and the monthly deposits on savings accounts.

To complete the household profile according to their assets ownership, the following indicators were considered: the possession of vehicles, radio, toaster, microwave, refrigerator, stove, washing machine, sewing machine, vacuum cleaner, domestic service, water availability, toilet, electricity, home ownership, water heater (gas and solar), and the monthly spending on household goods, vehicles acquisitions and home property (Table 1).

3.5   Index Estimation

The information related to income and expenses obtained from ENIGH was deflated in preparation for the analysis. Some new categorical variables were created to present the ownership of assets such as school loan, medical expenses insurance or life insurance. Some variables were converted from multi-level to binary to account only for the possession of the asset regardless of the number of items. A total of 49 variables were selected and gathered in a master dataset using the household folio number as the key in merging the different tables.

The package PCAmixdata [28] from R was applied to perform the mixed principal components analysis, and the dimensions and eigenvalues were obtained. The proportion of the total inertia explained by each dimension is used to determine the number of dimensions to keep.

The factor coordinates values of the dimensions selected are then used in the creation of the asset index, weighted by its own percentage of inertia explained (Eq. 3).

$$Y_i = \frac{x_{1i}w_1 + x_{2i}w_2 + \ldots + x_{ki}w_k}{w_1 + w_2 + \ldots + w_k} \tag{3}$$

Where Y_i is the value of the index for household i, x_{ki} is the value of the k factor coordinate selected, and w_i is the proportion of the total inertia explained by that coordinates. Finally, the value of Y_i is adjusted to a range between [0,100] to facilitate its interpretation. The asset index density distribution is estimated.

The index is used to compare Mexican households according to two attributes: their geographic location based on the state and its rural or urban condition. The mean and median of the value of the asset index per state is calculated, and this value is contrasted with the results of the Gini coefficient calculated on the same index per state.

The clustering k-mean method is used to identify the regions where Mexican households present low, medium, and higher levels of assets accumulation. The flowchart summarizing the process followed in the creation of the index is shown in Fig. 1.

Table 1. Variables selected for the analysis

Global Social Mobility Index Pillar	Variables selected from national survey of household income and expenditure	Type of variable
Health	Monthly spending in health Possession of medical expense insurance	Numerical Categorical (1 yes, 0 no)
Education access	Educational level of the head of household School loan	Categorical (from 1 to 11) Categorical (1 yes, 0 no)
Education quality and equity	Possession of scholarship Monthly scholarship received Monthly spending in education	Categorical (1 yes, 0 no) Numerical Numerical
Social protection	Retirement fund Access to "Seguro Popular" Affiliation for health care	Categorical (1 yes, 0 no) Categorical (1 yes, 0 no) Categorical (1 yes, 0 no)
Technology access	Telephone Cellular phone Pay TV Computer Printer Internet access Analog or Digital TV DVD or VCR Videogames Monthly spending in communications	Categorical (1 yes, 0 no) Categorical (1 yes, 0 no) Categorical (1 yes, 0 no) Categorical (1 yes, 0 no) Categorical (1 yes, 0 no) Categorical (1 yes, 0 no) Categorical (1 yes, 0 no) Categorical (1 yes, 0 no) Categorical (1 yes, 0 no) Numerical
Work opportunities	Own business Number of household members working and receive a salary	Categorical (1 yes, 0 no) Numerical
Working conditions	Written contract	Categorical (1 yes, 0 no)

Source: authors

4   Results

4.1   Asset Index Estimates

Based on the proportion of total inertia explained by each dimension, a total of 39 dimensions were selected accumulating 70.62% of proportion (Fig. 2). It is worth mentioning that discriminating some dimensions imply the loss of 29.38% of the variance of the information contained in the total dataset. However, this limitation is lessened by the fact that each of the dimensions maintained contains information on the total 49 variables selected.

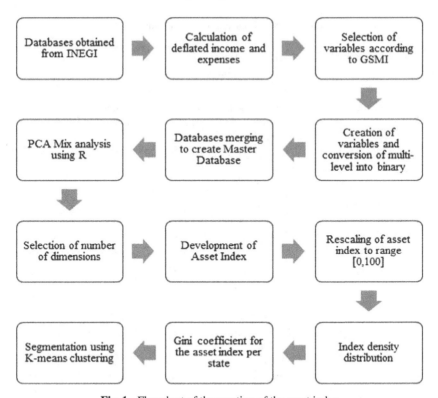

Fig. 1. Flowchart of the creation of the asset index

The coordinates corresponding to these first 39 dimensions were weighted by its own proportion of inertia and rescaled to create an asset index limited to values from 0 to 100.

The density distribution of the asset index calculated for the total households comprehended in the ENIGH survey shows a high right skewness, indicating high degree of inequality in the possession of assets among households (Fig. 3). Only 0.01% of the households possess 40% or more of the assets included in the index.

The main benefit obtained from the construction of the asset index comes from the additional disaggregated analysis that can be conducted. In the case of the Mexican households, the first analysis confirms that when separating rural and urban households, the distribution maintains the right skewness (Fig. 4).

Additionally, the index density was determined for each state. Even though the distribution shown in all states present the same skewed shape, the concentration of assets is higher in some states compared to others (Fig. 5).

The mean of the asset index for the entire sample of households contained in the survey is 6.93, which makes the skewness in the distribution even more evident, considering that the value ranges from 0 to 100. This number indicates that the average household in Mexico owns 6.93% of the total assets included in the index.

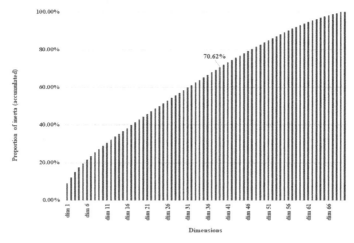

Fig. 2. Accumulated proportion of total inertia explained by each dimension

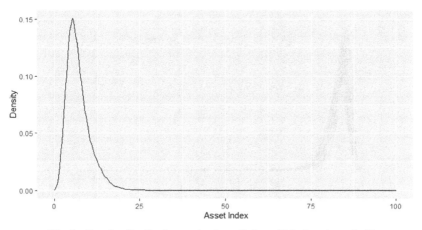

Fig. 3. Density distribution on the Asset Index of Mexican household

Segmenting households according to their rural or urban condition, it can be observed that urban households own a greater level of assets, but the disparity in the distribution is high in both conditions. In urban households, it is possible to find families possessing 100% of the assets included in the index, but at the same time families with indices as low as 0.08%. The median among urban households is 7.07, indicating that the asset possession level is low for most families (Table 2).

Contribution of the Assets to the Index (Loadings)
The contribution of each variable to each component (dimension) is called the loading. It can be observed that the first dimension is mostly influenced by assets related to technology (computer and internet access) and by the level of education of the household head. The second dimension presents a higher contribution from variables related to house

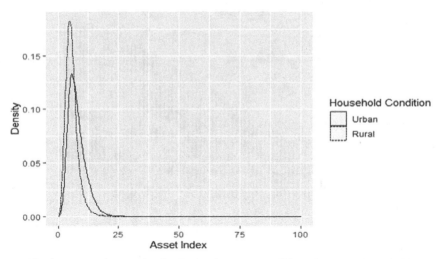

Fig. 4. Asset Index density distribution for urban condition of Mexican households

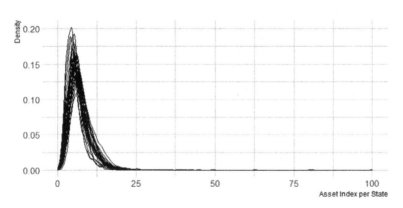

Fig. 5. Density distribution on the Asset index per Mexican states

Table 2. Descriptive statistics on the Asset Index according to Rural and Urban condition

	Mean	95% CI		Median	SD	Min	Max
		LL	UL				
Rural	5.63	5.6	5.66	5.26	2.68	0	80.58
Urban	7.73	7.7	7.77	7.07	3.68	0.08	100

Source: authors

ownership, and the sixth dimension shows a higher contribution form the possession of television (Table 3).

Here are presented only the most relevant variables contributing in the first ten dimensions, however, the asset index developed takes into consideration the contribution of all variables in the 39 dimensions kept. This is a variation compared to other indices created using standard PCA, where only the first component is taken. The methodology presented in this study creates the index as a weighted average of the contribution of the first 39 dimensions, and each dimension is at the same time computing different weights of contributions of the variables.

Table 3. Contribution of selected variables to the components (first ten dimensions)

Variable	dim 1	dim 2	dim 4	dim 5	dim 6	dim 7	dim 8	dim 10
Num. Members receive salary			0.418					
Monthly education expenses							**0.328**	
Scholarship							0.429	
Analog TV					0.664			
Digital TV					0.461			
Microwave	0.348							
Computer	0.430							
Monthly communic. expenses						**0.445**		
Internet access	0.467							
Education of household head	0.398							
Water	0.305							0.400
Electricity								
House ownership		0.700						
House loan		0.701		0.367				
Water heater (gas)	0.301							

Source: authors

An important aspect to highlight is that the variables that present the most important contributions to the components or dimensions include both categorical and numerical variables, reflecting the benefit of the method used. Had the standard PCA or MCA methods been used, the impact of the monthly expenses in education and communications would not have been considered because of its numerical nature -not categorical as most of the other variables are-.

The variables that are common among the households whose asset index is superior to 40 are the possession of cellular phone, water availability, electricity, computer, and particularly higher levels of education of the household head (graduate studies).

Index Concentration Degree by State

The asset index and the Gini Coefficient were contrasted for all 32 states. The asset index evaluates the ownership of assets among households, and therefore families will rank higher on the index if they own more assets. The Gini coefficient, on the other hand, measures the inequality in the distribution of assets among households. States with lower levels of Gini coefficient are those in which the distribution of assets is more equitable.

It can be observed the behavior of the Gini coefficient compared to the median of the asset index in every state, and it is mostly inverse. The decision of using the median in this comparison intends to reduce the impact of the extreme values of few households with higher asset indices (Fig. 6).

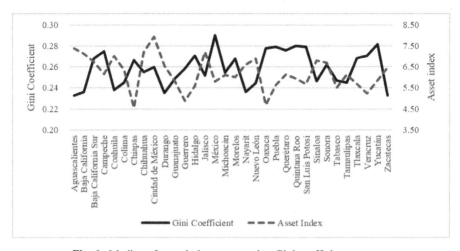

Fig. 6. Median of asset index compared to Gini coefficient per state

Ciudad de México is the state with the highest median of asset index, while Chiapas has the lowest. México State is the region where the distribution of assets is more unequal, while Zacatecas is the state with the most equitable distribution. However, this lower level of Gini coefficient is not always related to a higher ownership of assets; it could reflect regions inhabited by families with similar low or medium level of asset index.

Special attention must be taken to those states with the lowest level of asset possession that at the same time show high levels of concentration, because this inequality in the distribution of the assets may represent an obstacle for social mobility.

The comparison presented in Appendix 1 ranks the 32 states in ascending order according to their Gini coefficient and in descending order according to their asset index value using median and mean. Ciudad de México, the city capital of the country, ranks number one on the asset index but it ranks 17 according to the inequality of distribution. It is worth highlighting Aguascalientes that presents the second highest value of the median in the asset index, and it is also ranked second according to the values of the Gini coefficient, which indicates a state where the distribution of assets is more equitable, and households are able to own a higher number of these assets.

The Gini coefficient for rural households is 0.24 and for urban households is 0.25. Urban households own more assets than rural households, but at the same time they are more concentrated, that is, a less equitable distribution.

Disaggregation of the Index per State

The partition of groups of Mexican states using the k-mean clustering method was made based on the average asset index value of the households located in every state. Three clustering calculations were performed with 10, 5 and 3 clusters, and there was a drop in the intra-group sum of squares after every reduction in the number of clusters. The proportion of intra-group sum of squares of the total sum of squares dropped from 98.6% in a K(10) to 84.3% in K(3). Therefore, the analysis of the partitions of Mexican states is based on 3 groups (Fig. 7).

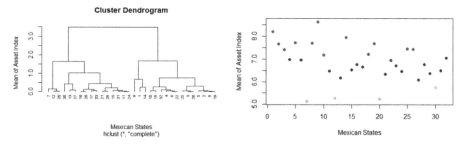

Fig. 7. Clustering of Mexican states according to the asset-index level

Four states belong to the group with the lowest level of asset accumulation, 16 states are in the medium-range group, and 12 states belong to the highest-level group. Cluster number one corresponds to the states with a low mean of asset index, and it groups Veracruz, Oaxaca, Guerrero and Chiapas. The states that form the Cluster number 2 are Baja California, Baja California Sur, Sonora, Chihuahua, Coahuila, Nuevo León, Sinaloa, Durango, Nayarit, Jalisco, Aguascalientes and Ciudad de México, and this group shows a high level of average asset index. Finally, Tamaulipas, San Luis Potosí, Zacatecas, Guanajuato, Querétaro, Colima. Michoacán, Estado de México, Hidalgo, Puebla, Morelos, Tlaxcala Tabasco, Campeche, Quintana Roo and Yucatán are the states grouped in the Cluster number 3, with medium level of asset index (Fig. 8).

When representing these clusters in the map, it is clear the difference in the three regions: the northern and western states as well as Ciudad de México belong to the group with the highest asset accumulation levels. The states located at the center and at the Yucatán Peninsula form the middle-range group, and the southern states of Oaxaca, Guerrero, Chiapas and Veracruz are the region where households own less assets.

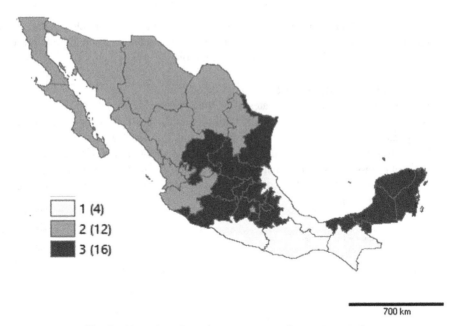

1 (4)
2 (12)
3 (16)

700 km

Fig. 8. Clustering of Mexican states according to Asset Index

5 Conclusions

A number of recent studies are using asset indices as alternative wealth measures when the information of other metrics such as income is not available, especially if the objective of the analysis is the evolution of the socio-economic status of households in different countries and different generations.

The index built in this study was estimated using the mixed principal components analysis, and presents some important differences compared to other indices aiming to evaluate socio-economic conditions:

1. Mixed principal components analysis allows the use of different types of variables: binary, categorical (multi-level) and numerical. This variety broadens the range of information that can be included in the index coming from surveys such as the national surveys of income and expenses, where not all variables are categorical.
2. An asset index that uses only categorical variables, particularly binary, would not include the simultaneous impact of the possession of a given asset (such as education) and the magnitude of the investment made by the household on that asset (measured by the amount of monthly expenses). The methodology used allows the inclusion of this simultaneous effect.

   Although these amounts are registered as expenses in the survey where the data is obtained from, they are considered in this study as assets since families benefit as they increase the monetary resources used in these activities.

3. Even though one of the main purposes of the method is the reduction of dimensions, each one of the dimensions selected for the integration of the index contain information of all the variables, lessening the negative effect of the loss of dimensions.
4. The weights assigned to every dimension and to every variable are not arbitrary. The dimensions are weighted by the proportion of the total inertia each dimension explains when they are averaged to compute the index. In addition, every dimension contains information of all the variables, showing a different proportion of contribution in every case. These proportions are derived from the correlations between the variable and the dimension.

The index was used in the evaluation of the how asset accumulation is distributed throughout the country and the degree of inequality in its distribution. The outcome show a clear segmentation of the Mexican states: northern states, western states and Ciudad de Mexico show the highest mean of asset index; center states and the Yucatan Peninsula region rank in the medium level; and southern states are those where the asset accumulation is the lowest.

The Gini Coefficient was useful to prove that regions where asset possession is lower, tend to present greater levels of inequality in its distribution. Southern states, thus, are the states where challenges for ascending social mobility are higher due to less availability of assets and greater levels of inequality.

These results are in line with other studies using wealth indices to measure inequality in the different Mexican regions [32], which shows the adequacy of the Mixed principal components analysis-based index in profiling the socioeconomic condition. Identifying the regions in which families have accumulated less assets allows the development of focalized policies intended to improve the access to different types of assets that are relevant for social mobility.

The methodology used in the present study is not restricted to the Mexican region. It can be useful in the development of asset indices in other countries where information of asset ownership, income and expenses at the household level is available.

Further analysis may use the asset index to measure intergenerational social mobility, overcoming the lack of sufficient income information from different generations. Other applications of this index may use it in the identification of the assets with highest impacts on social mobility and the probabilities of households to grow in their living conditions by possessing those assets.

Appendix 1. Comparison of Gini Coefficient and Mean and Median of the Asset Index of Mexican States

State	Gini Coef	State	Median of Index	State	Mean of Index
Zacatecas	0.23	Ciudad de México	7.93	Ciudad de México	8.63
Aguascalientes	0.23	Aguascalientes	7.39	Aguascalientes	8.19

(*continued*)

(*continued*)

State	Gini Coef	State	Median of Index	State	Mean of Index
Durango	0.24	Chihuahua	7.22	Jalisco	7.94
Nayarit	0.24	Jalisco	7.21	Coahuila	7.71
Baja California	0.24	Baja California	7.13	Chihuahua	7.69
Coahuila	0.24	Coahuila	7.02	Nuevo León	7.67
Nuevo León	0.24	Nuevo León	6.89	Baja California	7.66
Tamaulipas	0.24	Sinaloa	6.80	Sinaloa	7.45
Colima	0.24	Baja California Sur	6.76	Sonora	7.42
Sinaloa	0.25	Sonora	6.70	Baja California Sur	7.41
Tabasco	0.25	Nayarit	6.62	Nayarit	7.22
Guanajuato	0.25	Durango	6.56	Durango	7.18
Jalisco	0.25	Zacatecas	6.47	Zacatecas	7.05
Michoacán	0.25	Colima	6.35	Campeche	6.99
Chihuahua	0.25	Campeche	6.17	Colima	6.96
Guerrero	0.26	Querétaro	6.13	Querétaro	6.95
Ciudad de México	0.26	Tamaulipas	6.13	Michoacán	6.77
Sonora	0.26	Michoacán	6.10	Tamaulipas	6.76
Chiapas	0.27	Morelos	6.01	Quintana Roo	6.70
Baja California Sur	0.27	Quintana Roo	5.95	Morelos	6.65
Morelos	0.27	Yucatán	5.85	México	6.53
Tlaxcala	0.27	México	5.81	Yucatán	6.49
Hidalgo	0.27	Guanajuato	5.80	Guanajuato	6.48
Veracruz	0.27	San Luis Potosí	5.69	San Luis Potosí	6.46
Campeche	0.27	Tlaxcala	5.69	Tlaxcala	6.36
Querétaro	0.28	Puebla	5.64	Puebla	6.33
Oaxaca	0.28	Hidalgo	5.59	Hidalgo	6.18
San Luis Potosí	0.28	Tabasco	5.52	Tabasco	6.09
Puebla	0.28	Veracruz	5.23	Veracruz	5.74
Quintana Roo	0.28	Guerrero	4.87	Guerrero	5.28
Yucatán	0.28	Oaxaca	4.68	Oaxaca	5.25
México	0.29	Chiapas	4.55	Chiapas	5.14
Average	0.26	Average	6.20	Average	6.85

Source: authors with information from ENIGH 2018

Note. Gini index ordered in ascending order; mean and median ordered in descending order

References

1. Delajara, M., De la Torre, R., Díaz-Infante, E.: El México del 2018. Movilidad social para el bienestar. Centro de Estudios Espinosa Yglesias (2018)
2. Vélez-Grajales, R., Monroy-Gómez, L.A.: Movilidad social en México: hallazgos y pendientes. Revista de Economía Mexicana (2), 97–142 (2017)
3. Vélez-Grajales, R., Campos-Vázquez, R.M., Huerta-Wong, J.E.: Informe de movilidad social en México 2013: imagina tu futuro. CEEY Centro de Estudios Espinosa Yglesias, Ciudad de México (2013)
4. World Economic Forum: The global social mobility report 2020, Switzerland (2020)
5. Corak, M.: Income inequality, equality of opportunity, and intergenerational mobility. J. Econ. Perspect. **27**(3), 79–102 (2013)
6. Torche, F.: Changes in intergenerational mobility in Mexico: a cohort analysis. Centro de Estudios Espinosa Yglesias Documento de trabajo 03 (2020).
7. Behrman, J., Vélez-Grajales, V.: Patrones de movilidad intergeneracional para escolaridad, ocupación y riqueza en el hogar: el caso de México. In: Vélez-Grajales, H.W. (ed.) México, ¿el motor inmóvil?, pp. 299–346. CEEY Centro de Estudios Espinosa Yglesias, A.C., Ciudad de México (2015)
8. Vélez-Grajales, R., Vélez-Grajales, V., Stabridis, O.: Construcción de un índice de riqueza intergeneracional a partir de la encuesta ESRU de movilidad social en México (EMOVI). Centro de Estudios Espinosa Yglesias, Documento de trabajo 02/2015 (2015)
9. Vélez-Grajales, R., Stabridis Arana, O., Minor Campa, E.: Still looking for the land of opportunity: regional differences in social mobility in Mexico. Sobre México, Temas de Economía **1**, 54–69 (2018)
10. Sahn, D.E., Stifel, D.C.: Poverty comparisons over time and across countries in Africa. World Dev. **28**(12), 2123–2155 (2000)
11. Moser, C., Felton, A.: The construction of an asset index measuring asset accumulation in Ecuador. CPRC Vol. Working Paper 87 Washington DC: The Brookings Institution (2007)
12. Ferreira, F.H., Messina, J., Rigolini, J., López-Calva, L.-F., Lugo, M., Vakis, R.: La movilidad económica y el crecimiento de la clase media en América Latina. Banco Mundial, Washington, D.C (2013)
13. Inter-American Development Bank. La realidad social. Módulo 1 - Pobreza, Desigualdad y Movilidad Social (2020)
14. Vélez-Grajales, R., Campos-Vázquez, R., Fonseca, C.E.: El concepto de movilidad social: dimensiones, medidas y estudios en México. Centro de Estudios Espinosa Yglesias, Documento de trabajo (2015)
15. OCDE: A Broken Social Elevator? How to Promote Social Mobility. OECD Publishing, Paris (2018)
16. Cotler, P., Rodríguez-Oreggia, E.: Microfinanzas y la tenencia de activos no financieros en México. Investigación económica **69**(274), 63–86 (2010)
17. Filmer, D., Pritchett, L.: The effect of household wealth on educational attainment around the world: Demographic and health survey evidence. World Bank (1998)
18. Filmer, D., Pritchett, L.H.: Estimating wealth effects without expenditure data—or tears: an application to educational enrollments in states of India. Demography **38**, 115–132 (2001)
19. Sahn, D.E., Stifel, D.: Exploring alternative measures of welfare in the absence of expenditure data. Rev. Income Wealth **49**(4), 463–489 (2003)
20. Torche, F., Spilerman, S.: Influencias intergeneracionales de la riqueza en México. In: Serrano Espinosa, J., Torche, F. (eds.) Movilidad Social en México, población, desarrollo y crecimiento, pp. 229–274. Centro de Estudios Espinosa Yglesias, A.C., México (2010)

21. Asadullah, N.: Intergenerational economic mobility in rural Bangladesh. In: Royal Economic Society (RES) Annual Conference, Nottingham (2006)
22. Fajardo-Gonzalez, J.: Inequality of opportunity in adult health in Colombia. J. Econ. Inequal. **14**(4), 395–416 (2016). https://doi.org/10.1007/s10888-016-9338-2
23. Muhammad, M., Jamil, M.: Intergenerational mobility in educational attainments. Pak. Dev. Rev. **59**(2), 179–198 (2020)
24. Zeng, Z., Zhu, M.: Poverty groups identification and assessment of poverty alleviation programs in rural China. In: 6th International Conference on Humanities and Social Science Research, pp. 174–189. Atlantis Press (2020)
25. Rodriguez-Aguilar, R.: Main metric components in the generation of mixed indicators: an application of SGVD methodology. In: Vasant, P., Litvinchev, I., Marmolejo-Saucedo, J.A., Rodriguez-Aguilar, R., Martinez-Rios, F. (eds.) Data Analysis and Optimization for Engineering and Computing Problems. EICC, pp. 195–206. Springer, Cham (2020). https://doi.org/10.1007/978-3-030-48149-0_14
26. Beaton, D., Fatt, C.R.C., Abdi, H.: An ExPosition of multivariate analysis with the singular value decomposition in R. Comput. Stat. Data Anal. **72**, 176–189 (2014)
27. Kalantan, Z.I., Alqahtani, N.A.: A study of principal components analysis for mixed data. Int. J. Adv. Appl. Sci. **6**(12), 99–104 (2019)
28. Chavent, M., Kuentz-Simonet, V., Labenne, A., Saracco, J.: Multivariate analysis of mixed data: the R Package PCAmixdata. arXiv:1411.4911 (2017)
29. Flores, J.A.F., Gutiérrez, H.A., Zea, J.F.: Estimación por muestreo del índice de Gini para las localidades de Bogotá usando funciones en R. Comunicaciones en Estadística **8**(1), 59–79 (2015)
30. Handcock, M.S., Morris, M.: Relative Distribution Methods in the Social Sciences. Springer, Heidelberg (1999)
31. Morissette, L., Chartier, S.: The k-means clustering technique: general considerations and implementation in Mathematica. Tutor. Quant. Methods Psychol. **9**(1), 15–24 (2013)
32. Plassot, T., Rubio, G., Soloaga, I.: Movilidad social intergeneracional y desigualdad de oportunidades en México. Educación y activos: un enfoque territorial (2019)

Health Systems

A Data-Driven Study to Highlight the Correlations Between Ambient Factors and Emotion

Saeid Pourroostaei Ardakani[✉]🆔, Xinyang Liu, and Hongcheng Xie

School of Computer Science, University of Nottingham, Ningbo, China
{saeid.ardakani,scyxl6,scyhx1}@nottingham.edu.cn

Abstract. Emotion can be impacted by a variety of environmental or ambient factors. This means, people might show different affective reactions in response to ambient factors such as noise, temperature and humidity. Annoying ambient conditions (e.g., loud noise) may negatively influence people emotion and consequently address serious mental diseases. For this, ambient factors should be monitored and managed according to the users' preference to increase their statistician, enhance living experience quality and reduce mental-health risks. The purpose of this research is to study and predict the correlations between emotion and two ambient factors including temperature, and noise. For this, a system architecture is designed to measure user's affect in response to the indoor ambient factors. This system is tested in three experimental scenarios each of which with 15 participants. Ambient data is collected using an IoT enabled sensor network, whereas brainwaves are collected using an EEG. The brain signals are interpreted using a well-know API to recognise emotion state. Yet, two machine learning techniques KNN and DNN are used to analyse and predict emotional statues according to changing ambient temperature and noise. According to the results, DNN has a better accuracy to predict the emotional status as compared to KNN. Moreover, it shows that both noise and temperature are positively correlated to arousal and emotional status. Moreover, the results address that noise has a greater impact on emotion as compared to temperature.

Keywords: Emotion · Mental healthcare · Ambient factors · EEG

1 Introduction

Emotion is an innate and biological hardwired mechanism that promotes the survival of an organism by using adaptive responses to changing environmental circumstances [33]. This plays a crucial role in our life to respond to surrounding events. People may show different emotional statuses in various situations. For example, they feel happy when a new baby is born, excited to see a new place, or sad when they experience a break-up. However, emotion is different with

J. A. Marmolejo-Saucedo et al. (Eds.): COMPSE 2021, LNICST 393, pp. 109–128, 2021.
https://doi.org/10.1007/978-3-030-87495-7_8

mood. Emotion is a real-time reaction to the external events and it is usually short-term, whereas mood is the summary of the overall emotional states over a particular time period [29].

Emotional status can be recognised by behavioural, biological and/or brain signals [20]: (1) People show particular affective behaviours to respond to internal or external triggers/events [6]. For example, they might smile when they are happy or cry if they feel sad. This is difficult to recognise people affective behaviours as there is no unique behavioural emotion pattern and affective behaviours usually depend on a number of parameters such as culture, personality and/or gender [50], (2) Emotional status can be recognised using bio-signals. For example, heart-rate is increased if people are excited or surprised. However, bio-signal analysis is not able to accurately recognise emotional status as this can be influenced by a set of external factors such as illness, age and eating habits [18], (3) Brain signals (e.g., Alpha, Beta and/or Gamma signals) are measured by using Electroencephalogram (EEG) devices to recognise and study the emotional status [38]. However, this method is usually limited to experimental applications as the users have difficulty to wear EEG and feel unhappy to use it for long time.

Ambient conditions have the capacity to influence emotional statuses and address intuitive feelings, behaviours, habits or even health problems [28]. According to [54], environmental factors have the potential to address a varying degrees of behavioural problems, such as inattention, anger, and depression. This stems from the correlations of ambient factors/events and emotion and may address mental problems/issues as the results of human body's response to the surrounding environment [19]. For example, people might feel depressed or stressful if they stay in a dark room for a long time. Therefore, this is highly required to study the impact of environmental conditions on emotional statues to propose a particular correlation pattern. By this, people would be able to understand how to manage/control environmental factors such as light, noise, temperature and humidity to enhance affective experiences and mental-health conditions.

This paper aims to study the correlations between ambient factors (temperature and noise) and emotion. The key contribution of this research are outlined as below:

- Propose a data-driven experimental system architecture to collect and analyse ambient data (using an IoT enabled sensor network) and brainwaves (by using EEG).
- Test the accuracy of EEG device (EMOTIV EPOC+) and an brainwave enabled emotion recognition API by using a validated test dataset. This API is used to train and test the machine learning models which aim to predict emotional statues according to varying ambient parameters.
- Design and evaluate the performance of machine learning models in emotional status classification/prediction by using a real datasets collected from three experimental scenario each of which with 15 participants.

Under this research, three experimental scenarios including varying temperature, noise and temperature-noise are designed to study the impact of ambient factors on emotion. For this, an Internet of Things (IoT) enabled sensory system (AirRadio [1]) is deployed for ambient data collection, whereas a wearable wireless EEG equipment (named Emotiv EPOC+) is used to collect user's brain signals [45]. For each experimental scenario, brain signals are collected from 15 participants watching a (new)video while ambient conditions change. The sensory system captures and reports ambient data including temperature and noise via internet links. This research utilises a well-known emotion recognition API [42] to analyse EEG brainwaves and recognise/visualise emotional statues in real-time. The accuracy of the precensored API is tested by a validated online dataset, named SEED [61].

This paper takes the benefits of machine learning techniques -mainly K-Nearest Neighbour (KNN) [44] and Deep Neural Network (DNN) [27] to predict affective status influenced by ambient factors. The machine leaning models are trained and tested by using brainwaves collected from real participants who have been asked to wear the EEG while ambient conditions are changing. Self-descriptive questionnaires are collected to test and validate the accuracy of the proposed model.

The rest of this paper is structured as follow: Sect. 2 reviews the correlations of environmental factors and human emotion and mental-health. Section 3 introduces the research methodology and the proposed system architecture to collect and analyse recordings. Section 4 discusses the experimental results and highlights the research findings. Section 5 concludes the discussions and highlights the issues which still need to be addressed in the future.

2   Related Works

The relationship between emotion and (mental)health has attracted the attention of researchers during the past decades. Advances in the filed of affective computing allow us to analyse complex relationships between emotions, and external/internal factors such as environment and health [37]. Many studies have shown that physical symptoms often accompany emotional experiences [10]. This suggests that there might be a correlation between negative emotional statues and mental/physical health risks and diseases [31]. For example, negative emotions such as anger, anxiety and depression, may address serious cardiovascular diseases [51].

This is important to study the correlations of emotions and ambient factors to reduce/manage health risks. Positive emotions can significantly reduce the probability of stress and mental diseases such as depression [4], and thus improves mental health which has a great impact on family and society health and safety. In addition, many studies have shown that positive emotions address beneficial effects on general and physical health [46]. For example, this research [8] with an experimental sample size of 2000 participants over a period of 10 years reports a reduced 22% heart attacks ratio in positive emotion people. This supports that emotions have a high impact on people's mental and physical health.

2.1   EEG for Emotion Recognition

EEG is commonly used to collect brainwaves and recognise emotion. This captures and reports the brain neurons' voltage by using electrodes which measure the activities of multiple neurons in the brain cortex [45]. It usually measures frequencies ranging from 1 to 80 Hz with amplitudes ranging from 10 to 100 μV [22]. These signal frequencies are divided into different frequency bands, and certain frequency waves are more prominent in certain emotional states. The most important frequency waves are alpha (8–12 Hz), which is associated with brain inactivity, and beta (12–30 Hz), which is associated with active mental states [25].

The EEG signals are processed to extract emotional-related features, namely high/low arousal. For example, happiness is a state with high arousal, and the sadness is a state with low arousal [45]. However, the signals may still need to be filtered in advance to remove noise an enhance the signal quality.

Emotiv EPOC+ is one of the widely used EEG devices designed and released by Emotiv [16]. This head-mounted EEG device has 14 data collection electrodes that are positioned and tagged according to the standard of international 10–20 system [48]. As mentioned above, alpha and beta waves play a vital role in arousal measurement in emotion monitoring experiments and have the capacity to determine the level of brain activities. As [2] shows, AF3, AF4, F3 and F4 are the most commonly used locations for recording alpha and beta EEG signals in actual measurements. They are placed in the prefrontal cortex which plays a crucial role in emotion regulation. The electrodes monitor and measure the electrical signals and machine learning techniques are used to identify and predict emotional statues.

2.2   Machine Learning and Emotion Recognition

Machine learning (ML) techniques are increasingly being used to analyse, recognise and predict emotions. ML is used to analyse text and recognise the writer's emotional status. [49] takes the benefits of ML to categorize affective texts in children's books to achieve a better text-to-speech synthesis. This technology is used in teaching and learning applications to enhance the learning and students achievements as it has the capacity to emotionally engage students and teacher in learning [3]. Yet, ML can be used to recognise emotional statuses through behavioural cues such as facial expression [24]. Indeed, ML analyses and classifies the facial expressions/affective features which are captured/extracted using cameras.

ML techniques can be used to analyse brainwaves and recognise emotional cues. Brain signals are a key source to convey accurate cognitive and affective information [41]. They are divided into four waves according to their frequency: Delta, Theta, Alpha and Beta [57]. Brainwaves can form different emotional cues [55]. This addresses emotion recognition problem as a multi-category classification that should be resolved by using machine learning techniques. [14] analyses and compares a variety of machine learning techniques including Support Vector Machine (SVM) [17], K-nearest neighbour [44], Linear Discriminant Analysis [52], Logistic Regression [13] and Decision Trees [36].

[53] proposes two neural network models, namely simple deep and convolutional neural network, by using an EEG enabled dataset, called DEAP [53]. The results show that neural network can be an effective classifier for EEG signals, even more than the conventional machine learning techniques such as SVM.

[35] proposes an emotion prediction method combined with reinforcement learning. This is used to predict real-time emotional status during an online training to enhance the results of an online learning. It results in significant time reduction and achieves outstanding learning result and performance.

2.3   Environment and Emotion

Ambient factors include temperature, humidity, noise, light, and smell have the potential to influence people emotional statues. [11] studies the correlations of ambient noise on emotional statues. This aims to utilise a probability-based approaches to study the relationship between ambient factors and emotions. [23] reports that there is a close relationship between thermoregulation and emotion. According to this, environment temperature has an impact on the body regulation with a further impact on people's emotions [43] reports that higher temperatures significantly reduced happiness. Noise has the capacity to impact on emotion [7]. To support this, [40] addresses that loud noise negatively influence people emotion. Continuous high-volume sound treats mental health and may subject to harmful risks such as suicide. In addition, emotion can be influenced by ambient humidity [56]. This shows how humidity significantly impacts on students' happiness. Yet, ambient smell is taken into the account as an influential parameters on emotion. [9] shows environmental smells in public areas such as airport has the potential to affectively influence passengers.

The literatures address that a variety of ambient factors have the capacity to impact on mental health. Ambient conditions influence emotional statuses and consequently address mental health issues. There are a number of new and modern technologies to collect human brain wave data, and study how they are influenced by ambient factors such as noise, humidity and temperature. However, there is still a lack of applied research to analyse the correlations between ambient factors and emotions. This research utilises wearable EEG collection devices to collect emotional state changes of multiple participants in different environments, and use a variety of machine learning methods to highlight the specific correlations between ambient factors and emotions.

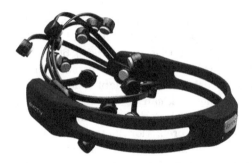

Fig. 1. EMOTIV EPOC+ device

3   Methodology

3.1   Experimental System Setup

This research proposes and deploys an experimental system architecture consisting of four key components including: ambient data collection, EEG data processing and analysis, self-feedback and machine leaning analysis.

An IoT enabled sensory network of AirRadio [1] devices is deployed to collect ambient data including temperature and noise. To manage the ambient conditions, small indoor cabins are equipped with air conditioner and Dolby speakers to change two ambient factors including ambient temperature and noise.

To analyse emotion, a wearable EEG equipment is used to collect and interpret user's brainwave. EMOTIV EPOC+ (Fig. 1 [16]) is one of the most widely-used low-cost wireless electroencephalography (EEG) [5]. It consists of 14 data-collection and 2 reference electrodes (AF3, F7, F3, FC5, T7, P7, 01, 02, P8, T8, FC6, F4, F8, AF4) that are labelled according to international 10–20 system of electrode placement [26]. Using EMOTIV EPOC+, five basic emotional states including happy, sad, fear, anger, surprise, and disgust are recognised.

Under this research, EMOTIV EPOC+ is used to collect brain signal for 15 participants who watch a video while changing ambient factors(temperature and noise). In turn, an open source and real-time emotion recognition API [42] is used to process and analyse the collected EEG data. This classifies input EEG dataset into five primary emotions including fear, happy, neutral, sad, relax according to the Russel's circumplex model of affect [47] and [62] (see Fig. 2).

To test the functionality, correctness and reliability of the emotion classification API, a validated online dataset, named SEED [61], is used. SEED dataset is an EEG dataset collected by Shanghai Jiao Tong University. This dataset contains EEG data from 15 groups of subjects, while watching affective videos labelled (based on arousal level) as negative, neutral and positive [32]. SEED is used to test the performance and accuracy of emotion recognition API. According to the results, this API is able to address an accuracy of 69.1% in emotion recognition. Yet, SEED is used to test the accuracy of EMOTIV EPOC+ EEG. For this, SEED data features are labelled according to EMOTIV EPOC+ channels and then the accuracy of emotion recognition is measured. According to our

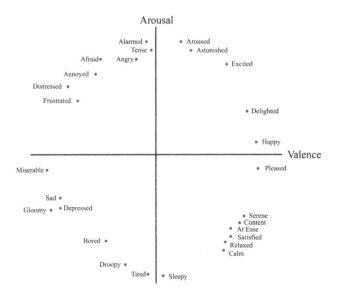

Fig. 2. Russell's circumplex emotion model

results, our EMOTIV EPOC+ is able to recognise correct emotional status with 72% accuracy.

A questionnaire is designed to collect user's self-describing experience and/or feedback at the end of each experiment. This allows to collect and analyse user feeling and recognise external factors -mainly background information which may influence the user's emotion and the experiment quality.

3.2 Experiment Design

This research aims to study the correlations between ambient factors-mainly temperature and noise and user emotion. Ambient factors are the research independent variables which change during each experiment, whereas emotion status is an dependent variable that is measured accordingly.

As Fig. 3 depicts, user data is collected in two forms: an online questionnaire and EEG. The former is a self-describing form to provide user's information and feeling during the experiments, whereas the latter collect user's brain signals to recognise the emotional status. User data is collected from 15 participants for each experiment. AirRadio sensor captures ambient data samples and forward the results to the system for aggregation and further analysis in real-time. The collected datasets are analysed and visualised to explore the correlations between ambient and affect data features. Yet, machine learning techniques including KNN and DNN are used to classify the predict the affect states according to ambient data change.

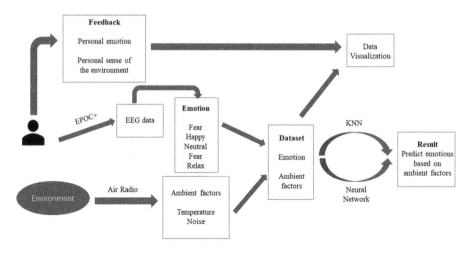

Fig. 3. The proposed experimental system architecture

To study the correlations between ambient factors and emotional status, three scenarios are designed. As Fig. 4 shows, the experimental scenarios (groups) are formed according to changing variables including (1) active temperature, as this changes while noise is fixed (no noise), (2) active noise, as it changes while temperature is fixed (standard indoor temperature), (3) active temperature and noise, both noise and temperature change. Each experiment includes 15 participants who participate in EEG data collection. They are asked to watch a documentary movie while ambient factors change. Each movie introduces a new and non-visited Chinese city in 10 min for each participant. This means, each participant watches a new city documentary that never visited or seen. Indeed, the participants are selected from a same age range 20–21 years old (male) and with no prior knowledge of the video content to minimise the impact of external parameters (e.g., gender, age and background knowledge) on the experimental results. As Fig. 7 and 9 show, ambient data including temperature and noise linearly change during each experiment and according to a particular range. This allows to study how people emotion changes if ambient noise and temperature change behind the comfort level (e.g., 20–22 centigrade degree for indoor temperature and 45–55 dB for indoor comfort acoustic level [30] and [12]). AirRadio sensor network reports ambient data samples each 10 s for aggregation and further analysis. At the same time, EEG data is collected from the participant with a 10-s time window for classification and analysis. KNN and DNN techniques are used to recognise the correlations between the ambient factors and emotional status. They are utilised to classify/predict the future emotional status according to ambient data changes.

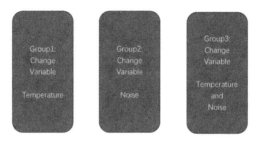

Fig. 4. Experimental scenarios

Machine Learning. This research utilises two machine learning technologies including k-nearest neighbours (KNNs) [44] and Deep neural network (DNN) [27] to analyse the collected EEG data, and predict the emotional statues corresponding to environmental conditions. For this, the experimental dataset is randomly partitioned into training (70%) and test (30%) datasets. Two machine learning models including to KNN and DNN are trained using the training dataset and used to label (predict the emotion value) test dataset. According to our results, the accuracy of KNN and DNN for emotion classification/prediction respectively are 71.19% and 74.57%. Hence, this is achieved that DNN has better precision performance to predict emotional status influenced by ambient factors as compared with KNN. Accuracy is calculated as the number of correct predictions over the total number of predictions.

KNN Machine Learning. Supervised learning is technique to extract the features of observed datasets to form an prediction model according to the application's objectives [34]. Indeed, supervisor learning utilises labelled data samples as a training datasets, and iteratively make predictions until the objectives are achieved [59]. There are two well-known supervised learning algorithms, linear support vector machines (SVM) [39] and k-nearest neighbours (KNN) [44], which are used in the literatures to study the correlations between datasets [21] and [2].

This research utilises k-nearest neighbours (KNN) [44] to classify emotional statuses and predict ambient-affect correlations. As Algorithm 1 shows, KNN recognises K nearest values (neighbours) in the dataset, and determines the most fitted emotion classes according to the value popularities [60]. For this, KNN machine learning model is proposed and trained to predict the affective status according to changing environmental factors. This addresses two phases: model training and test. For model training, the collected data from the users form a training dataset which is used to train KNN model. For the test phase, environmental factors are formed as the model's input, whereas five emotional states (fear, happy, sad, neutral and relax) are the machine learning model's output (classification labels).

Require:
  /*the coordinates of n training samples*/
  A[n];
  /*the nearest neighbour number*/
  k;
  /*new sample*/
  x;
Ensure:
  /*the class/label of x*/
  k_labels;
  /*initial k nearest neighbours of x*/
  A[1]~ A[k];
  /*Calculate the Euclidean distance between the test sample and x*/
  d(x, A[i]): i = 1, 2..., k;
  /*Sort d(x,A[i]) in ascending order*/
  Sort (d (x, A[i]));
  /*Calculate the distance D between the furthest sample and x*/
  D = Max (d (x, A[i]));

  /*Calculate the Euclidean distance between A[i] and x*/
  for $i = k + 1; i <= n; i + +$ **do**
    d (x, A[i]);
    if $d(x, A[i]) < D$ **then**
      Replace the farthest sample with A[i];
      /*Sort d(x,A[i]) in ascending order*/
      sort (d (x, A[i]));
      /*Calculate the distance D between the furthest sample and x*/
      D = Max (d (x, A[i]));
    end if
  end for

  /*Calculate the probability of first k samples belong to category*/
  k_labels = label (A[Top_k_index]);
  /*The class with greatest probability is the class of sample x*/
  Result = Max_prob(k_labels);

Algorithm 1: KNN Algorithm

Deep Neural Network. Deep neural network (DNN) [27] has the capacity to discover the coherence of input data features by adding an appropriate number of hidden layers to Feedforward Neural Networks. This uses a certain threshold value in output layer to address the label classifications. Neural network is an extension based on perceptron, while DNN is formed as a neural network with many hidden layers. Hence, DNN can be considered as a multilayer perceptron (neural network).

Multi-layer perceptron (MLP) [58] is a Feedforward artificial neural network model, which maps multiple input data sets to a single output data set. Hence,

MLP consists of nodes as multiple layers (input layer, hidden layer, and output layer) which are fully inter-connected. By this, MLP's forward propagation algorithm utilises the output of the previous layer to calculate the output of next layer. This uses several weight coefficient matrices (W) and bias (b) to carry out a series of linear and activation operations according to an input value vector (X). The calculation starts from the input layer, and sweeps the layers one-by-one until the output layer is reached and the result is calculated. The weight W and bias b are learned through back propagation. The objective is to minimize the difference between the predicted output and the expected output. For this, unknown input-output relationships are approximated by back propagating output layer errors into hidden layer [15].

This research proposes a network structure consisting of three layers: input layer, hidden layer and output layer. According to our results, three levels for hidden layers with 20 nodes work the best for this experimental plan. The input is the temperature and humidity of the 2 characteristic data environments, and the output is the 5 emotional categories (fear, happy, neutral, sad and relax). Figure 5 shows, the proposed DNN with three levels of hidden layers designed for the experiments.

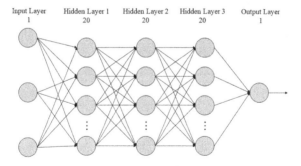

Fig. 5. Structure of DNN

4   Results and Discussion

This section discusses the experimental results to highlight the impact of ambient factors on emotional statues. According to experimental design, there are there categories for changing variables including noise, temperature, and temperature-noise. Each category aims to study the impact of the changing variable(s) on the emotional state. By this, the result of each category is presented to highlight the correlations of changing variables and emotional states. Figure 7 depicts temperature value is linearly reduced from 30.5 °C to 22 °C, whereas Fig. 9 shows how the noise level linearly changes during the experiment from 35 dB to 70 dB.

This research utilises data aggregation for data pre-processing and study the impact of ambient factors on emotional status. For this, a time-based Average aggregation function is used for environmental data to calculate the average of each ambient value from each experiment cabin (user indoor area) according to a particular timing plan (10 min experiment). Emotional statues are aggregated according to a Mode function. For this, emotional statues of each user are collected and listed as a vector. In turn, a mode value is calculated to update the dataset and machine leaning model training [62].

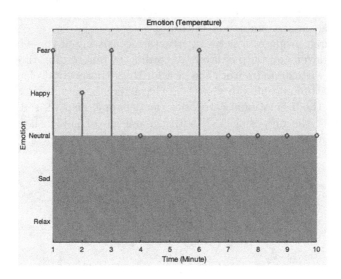

Fig. 6. Mode of participants' emotional statues (varying temperature)

4.1 Varying Temperature

As Fig. 6 shows, user emotional status can be influenced by indoor temperature. In other words, the users are emotionally behave to do a particular task if indoor temperature changes during the experiments. The participants start the experiment with a particular psychological state (e.g., fear as (mode)emotional state for the majority of participants). This stems from the fact that they feel strange to join a new experiment in which they should watch an unseen video of an unknown city. Yet, they may feel uncomfortable due to the high indoor temperature as Fig. 7 shows. However, the participants' emotional states change (fear to happy) and they gradually become neutral for a while (until 6) as they fully engaged with the movie, adapted to the experiment and environment and the temperature meets the indoor comfort level. This supports that the participants feel happy when they feel safe and convenience after several minutes watching a video where indoor temperature is not high.

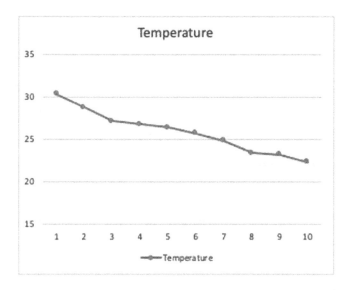

Fig. 7. Temperature chart

According to the results, this is found that emotional statues become happy (low-aroused) and/or neutral (no-aroused) when the ambient temperature drops from high to more comfortable values. This means, people feel uncomfortable and experience high-aroused emotional status such as fear when the temperature is high such as 30 °C. However, their affective status will become happy and then neutral if the temperature gradually decreases and meets the indoor comfort level. According to Fig. 6, indoor thermal comfort level rage [30] is supported and the participants experience happy and neutral emotional state when indoor temperature meets the comfort level 22 to 24 °C.

4.2   Varying Noise

According to Fig. 8, there is a certain relationship between the environmental noise and the participants' emotional state and the participants are emotionally influenced by varying noise. As the result show, participants mostly experience happy emotional status during the first minutes of the experiment when there is no or low level of noise. However, they feel affectively aroused-mainly fear if ambient noise is increased. They feel neutral and there is no significant affective change for a while when the noise level meets the acoustic comfort level (45–55 dB) and the participants are adapted to the ambient nose level. However, they feel aroused and feared again when the ambient noise level is significantly increased and reached around 70 dB.

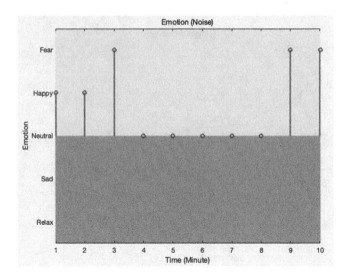

Fig. 8. Mode of participants' emotional statues (varying noise)

As results show, the participants experience aroused-emotion such as fear when the noise is suddenly increased. The emotional states are gradually changed to neutral if they are adapted to the ambient noise which is slowly increased. However, they feel fear and/or highly aroused when the noise level is highly increased and reaches around 70 dB. This supports that high-level noise (e.g., 70 dB) is annoying, addresses high-aroused emotion such as fear [28].

4.3 Varying Temperature and Noise

Simultaneous changing ambient factors has the capacity to influence users' emotions. As Fig. 10 shows, the participants' emotional statues are influenced if both temperature and noise change at the same time. During the experiment, both the ambient parameters gradually change while the participants run experiment and watch the video. Temperature is reduced from 30 °C to 22 °C, whereas ambient noise is increased from 35 dB to 70 dB. According to the results, the mode of participants emotional statues remains neutral and/or sad (low arousal) during the first two minutes of the experiments. In other words, the majority of the participants experience sad emotion when the temperature is decreased into indoor comfort level and noise is increased. The results show a similar emotional behaviour and the participants feel neutral (or sad) if the temperature is decreased to meet indoor comfort level, but the increasing noise is still in a standard level. However, they feel aroused (e.g., fear) when the noise level is highly increased (70 dB) and annoys them during the experiments. They feel fear even indoor temperature meets comfort level. This means, noise has a greater impact on emotion as compared to temperature.

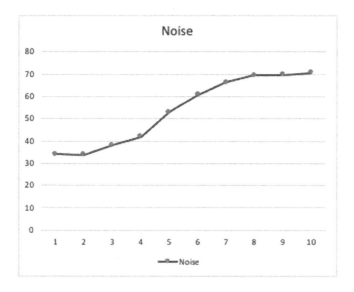

Fig. 9. Noise chart

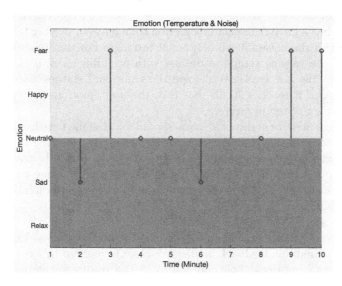

Fig. 10. Mode of participants' emotional statues (varying temperature and noise)

5   Conclusion and Further Work

This research focuses on a data-driven study to highlight the impact of ambient factors on emotional status. This has the capacity to offer mental healthcare teams a number of benefits to understand how emotion is influenced by varying ambient factors. Indeed, this research highlights the impact of ambient conditions on people affective behaviour when they respond to changing environment while doing a particular task such as watching a video. Under this research, EMOTIV EPOC+ EEG is used to collect brain signals from three experimental scenarios including varying temperature, noise and temperature-noise. 15 participants join each experimental scenario to wear the EEG and watch a never-seen documentary movie for 10 min. The EEG collects brainwaves are measured using (labelled) electrodes to recognise five basic emotional statuses (Neutral, Happy, Sad, Fear and Relax). At the same time, a sensory system (AirRadio) collects and reports real-time ambient data including temperature and noise. The collected ambient data is used to study how they influence emotional statuses. This research utilises KNN and DNN to analyse and predict emotional status according to the ambient variables. DNN works better when the hidden layer is set as 3 layer, and the nodes are 20. According to the results, 71.19% and 74.57% of accuracy are respectively achieved for KNN and DNN learning predictions.

The experimental results support and highlight the correlation of environmental data and emotion. None or limited increased arousal (neutral or happy) is observed if the ambient temperature is decreased form high to meet indoor comfort level, whereas people experience high aroused emotional statues when environment becomes hot. Yet, the participants feel feared and high aroused when the ambient noise become annoying (over 70 dB). According to the results, temperature has a greater impact on emotion than noise in varying temperature-noise scenario if the noise (30–65 dB) is not too high. For this, emotion changes according to the varying temperature and with no influence of noise. However, noise becomes the key reason to change the emotional statues and makes the people aroused if it reaches 70 dB. For this, the user emotionally experiences a minimum impact of temperature.

In future, a new experimental plan should be designed with an increased number of tasks during a longer experiment time. By this, the experimental dataset includes a greater number of data features to highlight the impact of ambient factors on emotion. Indeed, this allows machine learning techniques to form a more accurate prediction model which supports a greater number of states per each action.

Wearable sensory devices such as Galvanic Skin Response (GSR) can be used in the future to enhance the accuracy of emotional recognition. This helps to measure the human bio-feedback in affective cases influenced by external factors such as ambient conditions. This may returns better results as compared to EEG because bio-feedback sensors usually are easier to wear and carry.

The impact of ambient factors such as occupancy and pollution on emotional status also can be addressed as future work. The ambient factors should be collected using a sensor network to report the air pollution and real-time occupancy. At the same time, brain signals should be recorded to observe how they change according to the variety of the ambient factors.

References

1. AirRadio (2021). https://www.desertcart.com.kw/products/61155735-air-radio-a-2-se-pm-2-5-pm-10-detector-humidity-temperature-sensor-air-quality-monitor. Accessed January 2021
2. Aldayel, M., Ykhlef, M., Al-Nafjan, A.: Deep learning for EEG-based preference classification in neuromarketing. Appl. Sci. **10**(4), 1525 (2020). https://doi.org/10.3390/app10041525
3. Altrabsheh, N., Cocea, M., Fallahkhair, S.: Predicting students' emotions using machine learning techniques. In: Conati, C., Heffernan, N., Mitrovic, A., Verdejo, M.F. (eds.) AIED 2015. LNCS (LNAI), vol. 9112, pp. 537–540. Springer, Cham (2015). https://doi.org/10.1007/978-3-319-19773-9_56
4. Ardakani, S.P.: MSAS: an M-mental health care system for automatic stress detection. Clin. Psychol. Stud. **7**, 72–80 (2017). https://doi.org/10.22054/jcps.2017.8156
5. Badcock, N.A., Mousikou, P., Mahajan, Y., De Lissa, P., Thie, J., McArthur, G.: Validation of the Emotiv EPOC® EEG gaming system for measuring research quality auditory ERPS. PeerJ **1**, e38 (2013)
6. Balconi, M., Fronda, G., Venturella, I., Crivelli, D.: Conscious, pre-conscious and unconscious mechanisms in emotional behaviour. Some applications to the mindfulness approach with wearable devices. Appl. Sci. **7**(12), 1280 (2017)
7. Biswas, D., Lund, K., Szocs, C.: Sounds like a healthy retail atmospheric strategy: effects of ambient music and background noise on food sales. J. Acad. Mark. Sci. **47**(1), 37–55 (2019)
8. Boehm, J.K., Kubzansky, L.D.: The heart's content: the association between positive psychological well-being and cardiovascular health. Psychol. Bull. **138**(4), 655 (2012)
9. Bogicevic, V., Yang, W., Cobanoglu, C., Bilgihan, A., Bujisic, M.: Traveler anxiety and enjoyment: the effect of airport environment on traveler's emotions. J. Air Transp. Manag. **57**, 122–129 (2016)
10. Carter, L., Ogden, J.: Evaluating interoceptive crossover between emotional and physical symptoms. Psychol. Health Med. **26**, 1–10 (2020)
11. Choi, S.G., Cho, S.B.: Bayesian networks+ reinforcement learning: controlling group emotion from sensory stimuli. Neurocomputing **391**, 355–364 (2020)
12. Craig, A.: A new view of pain as a homeostatic emotion. Trends Neurosci. **26**(6), 303–307 (2003)
13. Cramer, J.: The origins of logistic regression. SSRN Electron. J. (2003). https://doi.org/10.2139/ssrn.360300
14. Doma, V., Pirouz, M.: A comparative analysis of machine learning methods for emotion recognition using EEG and peripheral physiological signals. J. Big Data **7**(1), 1–21 (2020)
15. Durairaj, M., Revathi, V.: Prediction of heart disease using back propagation MLP algorithm. Int. J. Sci. Technol. Res. **4**(8), 235–239 (2015)
16. Emotiv: Emotiv EPOC+ (2021). https://www.emotiv.com/epoc/. Accessed January 2021
17. Evgeniou, T., Pontil, M.: Support vector machines: theory and applications. In: Paliouras, G., Karkaletsis, V., Spyropoulos, C.D. (eds.) ACAI 1999. LNCS (LNAI), vol. 2049, pp. 249–257. Springer, Heidelberg (2001). https://doi.org/10.1007/3-540-44673-7_12
18. Goshvarpour, A., Abbasi, A., Goshvarpour, A.: Influence of age and gender on emotional skin response. Int. J. Psychol. (IPA) **11**(2), 126–151 (2017)

19. Gruebner, O., Rapp, M.A., Adli, M., Kluge, U., Galea, S., Heinz, A.: Cities and mental health. Dtsch. Arztebl. Int. **114**(8), 121 (2017)

20. Hamada, M., Zaidan, B., Zaidan, A.: A systematic review for human EEG brain signals based emotion classification, feature extraction, brain condition, group comparison. J. Med. Syst. **42**(9), 1–25 (2018)

21. Hastie, T., Tibshirani, R., Friedman, J.: The Elements of Statistical Learning. Springer Series in Statistics, Springer, New York (2009). https://doi.org/10.1007/978-0-387-84858-7

22. Hudspeth, A.J., Jessell, T.M., Kandel, E.R., Schwartz, J.H., Siegelbaum, S.A.: Principles of Neural Science. McGraw-Hill, Health Professions Division, New York (2013)

23. IJzerman, H., Heine, E.C., Nagel, S.K., Pronk, T.M.: Modernizing relationship therapy through social thermoregulation theory: evidence, hypotheses, and explorations. Front. Psychol. **8**, 635 (2017)

24. Jain, D.K., Shamsolmoali, P., Sehdev, P.: Extended deep neural network for facial emotion recognition. Pattern Recogn. Lett. **120**, 69–74 (2019)

25. Jebelli, H., Hwang, S., Lee, S.: EEG signal-processing framework to obtain high-quality brain waves from an off-the-shelf wearable EEG device. J. Comput. Civ. Eng. **32**(1), 04017070 (2018)

26. Jeon, S., Chien, J., Song, C., Hong, J.: A preliminary study on precision image guidance for electrode placement in an EEG study. Brain Topogr. **31**(2), 174–185 (2018)

27. Jirayucharoensak, S., Pan-Ngum, S., Israsena, P.: EEG-based emotion recognition using deep learning network with principal component based covariate shift adaptation. Sci. World J. **2014** (2014)

28. Kanjo, E., Younis, E.M., Sherkat, N.: Towards unravelling the relationship between on-body, environmental and emotion data using sensor information fusion approach. Inf. Fusion **40**, 18–31 (2018)

29. Kaplan, R.L., Levine, L.J., Lench, H.C., Safer, M.A.: Forgetting feelings: opposite biases in reports of the intensity of past emotion and mood. Emotion **16**(3), 309 (2016)

30. Karmann, C.: Thermal comfort and acoustic quality in buildings using radiant systems. Ph.D. thesis, Architecture Department, University of California, Berkeley (2017)

31. Kunzmann, U., Wrosch, C.: Comment: the emotion-health link: perspectives from a lifespan theory of discrete emotions. Emot. Rev. **10**(1), 59–61 (2018)

32. Lan, Z., Sourina, O., Wang, L., Scherer, R., Müller-Putz, G.R.: Domain adaptation techniques for EEG-based emotion recognition: a comparative study on two public datasets. IEEE Trans. Cogn. Dev. Syst. **11**(1), 85–94 (2018)

33. Levenson, R.W., Lwi, S.J., Brown, C.L., Ford, B.Q., Otero, M.C., Verstaen, A.: Emotion. In: Handbook of Psychophysiology, pp. 444–464. Cambridge University Press (2017). https://doi.org/10.1017/9781107415782.020

34. Liu, B.: Supervised learning. In: Web Data Mining. Data-Centric Systems and Applications, pp. 63–132. Springer, Heidelberg (2011). https://doi.org/10.1007/978-3-642-19460-3_3

35. Liu, W., Zhang, L., Tao, D., Cheng, J.: Reinforcement online learning for emotion prediction by using physiological signals. Pattern Recogn. Lett. **107**, 123–130 (2018)

36. Maimon, O., Rokach, L.: Data Mining and Knowledge Discovery Handbook. Springer, Boston (2005). https://doi.org/10.1007/b107408D

37. Marín-Morales, J., et al.: Affective computing in virtual reality: emotion recognition from brain and heartbeat dynamics using wearable sensors. Sci. Rep. **8**(1), 1–15 (2018)
38. Mehmood, R.M., Du, R., Lee, H.J.: Optimal feature selection and deep learning ensembles method for emotion recognition from human brain EEG sensors. IEEE Access **5**, 14797–14806 (2017)
39. Meyer, D., Wien, F.T.: Support vector machines. The Interface to LIBSVM in package **28**, e1071 (2015)
40. Min, J.Y., Min, K.B.: Night noise exposure and risk of death by suicide in adults living in metropolitan areas. Depress. Anxiety **35**(9), 876–883 (2018)
41. Moon, S.E., Jang, S., Lee, J.S.: Convolutional neural network approach for EEG-based emotion recognition using brain connectivity and its spatial information. In: 2018 IEEE International Conference on Acoustics, Speech and Signal Processing (ICASSP), pp. 2556–2560. IEEE (2018)
42. nadzeri: Realtime-EEG-based-emotion-recognition (2016). https://github.com/nadzeri/Realtime-EEG-Based-Emotion-Recognition. Accessed January 2021
43. Noelke, C., et al.: Increasing ambient temperature reduces emotional well-being. Environ. Res. **151**, 124–129 (2016)
44. Peterson, L.E.: K-nearest neighbor. Scholarpedia **4**(2), 1883 (2009)
45. Ramirez, R., Vamvakousis, Z.: Detecting emotion from EEG signals using the emotive EPOC device. In: Zanzotto, F.M., Tsumoto, S., Taatgen, N., Yao, Y. (eds.) BI 2012. LNCS (LNAI), vol. 7670, pp. 175–184. Springer, Heidelberg (2012). https://doi.org/10.1007/978-3-642-35139-6_17
46. Revord, J., Sweeny, K., Lyubomirsky, S.: Categorizing the function of positive emotions. Curr. Opin. Behav. Sci. **39**, 93–97 (2021)
47. Russell, J.A.: A circumplex model of affect. J. Pers. Soc. Psychol. **39**(6), 1161–1178 (1980). https://doi.org/10.1037/h0077714
48. Schomer, D.L., Da Silva, F.L.: Niedermeyer's Electroencephalography: Basic Principles, Clinical Applications, and Related Fields. Lippincott Williams & Wilkins (2012)
49. Sinclair, J.: Using machine learning to predict children's reading comprehension from lexical and syntactic features extracted from spoken and written language. Ph.D. thesis, University of Toronto, Canada (2020)
50. de Souza, L.C., et al.: The effects of gender, age, schooling, and cultural background on the identification of facial emotions: a transcultural study. Int. Psychogeriatr. **30**(12), 1861 (2018)
51. Suls, J.: Toxic affect: are anger, anxiety, and depression independent risk factors for cardiovascular disease? Emot. Rev. **10**(1), 6–17 (2018)
52. Tharwat, A., Gaber, T., Ibrahim, A., Hassanien, A.E.: Linear discriminant analysis: a detailed tutorial. AI Commun. **30**(2), 169–190 (2017)
53. Tripathi, S., Acharya, S., Sharma, R.D., Mittal, S., Bhattacharya, S.: Using deep and convolutional neural networks for accurate emotion classification on DEAP dataset. In: Proceedings of the Thirty-First AAAI Conference on Artificial Intelligence, pp. 4746–4752 (2017)
54. Veenstra, L., Koole, S.L.: Disarming darkness: effects of ambient lighting on approach motivation and state anger among people with varying trait anger. J. Environ. Psychol. **60**, 34–40 (2018)
55. Wang, K.J., Zheng, C.Y.: Toward a wearable affective robot that detects human emotions from brain signals by using deep multi-spectrogram convolutional neural networks (deep MS-CNN). In: 2019 28th IEEE International Conference on Robot and Human Interactive Communication (RO-MAN), pp. 1–8. IEEE (2019)

56. Wells, V.K., Daunt, K.L.: Eduscape: the effects of servicescapes and emotions in academic learning environments. J. Furth. High. Educ. **40**(4), 486–508 (2016)

57. Yang, H.W., Lin, J.S., Hwang, M.S.: Research and development of brainwave recognition technology and its access control application. Int. J. Electron. Inf. Eng. **12**(3), 136–145 (2020)

58. Zhang, C., et al.: A hybrid MLP-CNN classifier for very fine resolution remotely sensed image classification. ISPRS J. Photogramm. Remote. Sens. **140**, 133–144 (2018)

59. Zhang, M.L.: A k-nearest neighbor based multi-instance multi-label learning algorithm. In: 2010 22nd IEEE International Conference on Tools with Artificial Intelligence, vol. 2, pp. 207–212. IEEE (2010)

60. Zhang, S., Li, X., Zong, M., Zhu, X., Cheng, D.: Learning k for kNN classification. ACM Trans. Intell. Syst. Technol. (TIST) **8**(3), 1–19 (2017)

61. Zheng, W.L., Lu, B.L.: Investigating critical frequency bands and channels for EEG-based emotion recognition with deep neural networks. IEEE Trans. Auton. Ment. Dev. **7**(3), 162–175 (2015)

62. Zhong, K., Qiao, T., Zhang, L.: A study of emotional communication of emoticon based on Russell's circumplex model of affect. In: Marcus, A., Wang, W. (eds.) HCII 2019. LNCS, vol. 11583, pp. 577–596. Springer, Cham (2019). https://doi.org/10.1007/978-3-030-23570-3_43

Telerehabilitation Prototype for Postural Disorder Monitoring in Parkinson Disease

Jorge L. Rojas-Arce[1] (ID), Luis Jimenez-Angeles[1](✉) (ID),
and Jose Antonio Marmolejo-Saucedo[2] (ID)

[1] Departamento de Ingenieria en Sistemas Biomedicos, Facultad de Ingenieria, Universidad Nacional Auonoma de Mexico, Mexico City, Mexico
{jorge.rojas.arce,luis.jimenez}@comunidad.unam.mx
[2] Facultad de Ingenieria, Universidad Panamericana, Augusto Rodin 498, 03920 Mexico City, Mexico
jmarmolejo@up.edu.mx

Abstract. The present work shows a telerehabilitation prototype for the monitoring of postural disorders in patients with Parkinson's disease. The design of this prototype originated from a proposal for the identification of business ideas in medical devices. Specifically, the steps that were followed were to detect a need, formulate hypotheses about the problem and the client who faces them in their day-to-day life, then validate them through interviews with clients, to formulate the hypothesis of the solution; and build a prototype that offers value and solves previously detected needs. This prototype allows to make measurements, and eventually corrections of the postures in patients with Parkinson's disease, using devices that can be used remotely as part of the interaction between the doctor and the patient.

Keywords: Telerehabilitation · Parkinson's disease · Business ideas

1 Introduction

The pandemic has accelerated the adoption of tele-health in many countries. In the US, according to Fair Health, the usage of tele-health has increased over 4,300% between March 2019 and March 2020.

When the pandemic will be over many of the services (like prescriptions) will be delivered from remote. Figure 1 shows with the black bar the amount of tele-consultations in 2019 (in %) versus the amount of tele-consultations expected in the post pandemic phase [1].

Tele-health is disrupting the geography of health care. In the coming years we may see the rise of points of excellence providing this service to people all over the world. This tele-service provisioning is bound to create hubs of delivery and the management of the increasing demand will be met, most likely, with automatic response systems, software applications based on artificial intelligence, plus a systematic use of natural language interaction.

© ICST Institute for Computer Sciences, Social Informatics and Telecommunications Engineering 2021
Published by Springer Nature Switzerland AG 2021. All Rights Reserved
J. A. Marmolejo-Saucedo et al. (Eds.): COMPSE 2021, LNICST 393, pp. 129–142, 2021.
https://doi.org/10.1007/978-3-030-87495-7_9

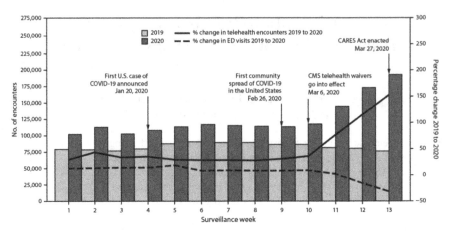

Fig. 1. Figures indicating the usage of tele-health services in the US.

Each patient will have a corresponding healthcare record, recording his vitals (possibly automatically updated in quasi-real time depending on the level of service required), prescriptions taken, plus all the result of exams, consultations and the sequence of his genome. This record will be used by machine learning algorithms to create a model of that person and a variety of software applications will be monitoring both the patient and the potential risk of the environment on that patient. In other words, this shift towards tele-health will be supported, and mediated, by the creation and use of personal digital twins.

Additionally, the delivery of healthcare support, particularly monitoring, using software and personal digital twins can enable continuous consultation (one person may get in touch with her virtual doctor as many times as wished, every single day with a single subscription cost. The increased effort on the provider side is negligible, the perceived advantage on the receiving side is huge. As an additional benefit, the more a person uses the service the more data are being accrued, increasing the provider data space value [1].

The Parkinson's Disease (PD) is a neurological disorder with an overall prevalence of 0.3%, increasing up to more than 3% in the population above 80 years old, and an incidence estimated to range between 5 to 35 cases per 100'000 individuals each year [1]. Its three cardinal motor symptoms are bradykinesia, resting tremor and rigidity, which is clinically defined as the increased resistance in response to the passive motion of joints [2].

In the case of Mexico, the medical device industry is changing, because of new research topics and technological advances related to health. However, there is a situation that, in many cases, is not considered, such as the interaction of users with said devices, which in many cases is limited to obtaining only certain information about health, and/or, when they offer a treatment (therapy) that is only limited to already defined movements, which, in many cases, are not those specifically required by the user.

A medical device is an instrument, apparatus, utensil, machine, including the software for its operation, implantable product or material, diagnostic agent, material, substance or similar product, to be used, alone or in combination, directly or indirectly in beings' humans; with any of the following purposes of use [3].

- Diagnosis, prevention, surveillance, or monitoring, and/or assisting in the treatment of diseases.
- Diagnosis, surveillance or monitoring, treatment, protection, absorption, drainage, or aid in the healing of an injury.
- Substitution, modification or support of the anatomy or a physiological process.
- Life support.
- Control of conception.
- Disinfection of Medical Devices.
- Disinfectant substances.
- Provision of information through an in vitro examination of Samples extracted from the human body, for diagnostic purposes.
- Devices that incorporate tissues of animal and/or human origin, and/or
- Devices used in in vitro fertilization and assisted reproductive technologies.

Hand in hand with knowing the impact of technology, it is also necessary to identify a specific real problem related to the use of technology, from a technical point of view to a commercial aspect. Therefore, entrepreneurial processes to find something that does not yet have a solution or something that has an inappropriate solution is a starting point to talk about business [4]. In fact, in the case of Parkinson's Disease, an assessment of rigidity in an unstructured environment has been poorly investigated since it is hard to achieve with instrumentation currently available [2].

Specifically, in this work is presented a proposal to solve the problem of design, build and put in market many medical devices, whose they are no accepting and buying for patients. The origin of problem to be solved is how to identify business ideas in medical devices.

A methodology is proposed for this problem, which begins with the detection of a need on patients, a hypothesis is formulated about that need and how the patient faces them in their day to day, and then validates them through interviews whomselves. Once validated, a solution hypothesis is formulated; and a prototype is built that offers value and solves patient needs that were previously detected.

To test this proposal, a practical application of this proposal is presented, which shows the generation of a prototype that allows access to a rehabilitation teletherapy, using devices for remote monitoring of the movement of patients with the disease of Parkinson. In the development of this proposal, the online collaboration between the project team and the medical support staff stands out, as well as the online collection of patient information.

2 Methodology

The proposal presented here shows how to establish a business idea with a high probability of commercial success, since it presents an initial validation that is done with the potential users or clients of the solution proposal that is being presented. This proposal consists of the following steps: detection of a need; formulation of a hypothesis about the problem and the client; validation of the hypothesis of the problem and the client regarding this detected need; formulation of the hypothesis of the solution; and finally, construction of a prototype that offers value to customers, solving previously detected needs. Each of these parts is presented in detail below and put into practice with the case study of patients with Parkinson's disease.

2.1 Detection of a Need

It begins with the detection of a need that motivates the development of a business idea. Specifically, this need is contextualized in the knowledge and experience that the proponent has about the environment where the detection was made. And in the same way, before the detection of this need, a business idea will arise that shows a solution for it.

To show the detection of the need, the storyboard tool [5] was used, which graphically shows how a problematic situation (need) that some customers are suffering is presented and how it is that from a proposed solution a solution is given to this need.

Figure 2 shows how the need was detected for a patient with Parkinson's disease.

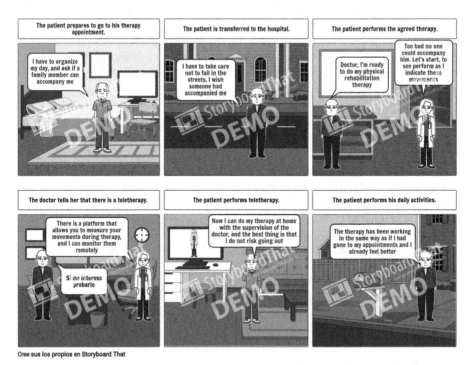

Cree sus los propios en Storyboard That

Fig. 2. Figures indicating a proposed solution for Parkinson's patients (storyboard created with the tool www.storyboardthat.com).

As can be seen in Fig. 2 (a)–(c), the daily life of a patient with Parkinson's disease is affected in the performance of their daily activities and is further aggravated by having to move to their therapies in medical institutions. Emphasis is placed on the difficulty of having to move to therapies and in performing therapies under the supervision of the doctor for their proper performance. In turn, Figs. 2 (d)–(e) also show a first approach of what a solution would look like, through a platform that allows physical rehabilitation therapy to be carried out at a distance, with the supervision of a specialist doctor.

2.2   Formulation of a Hypothesis About the Problem and the Client

The next step is to formulate the hypotheses of what is the problem that the clients face, and in turn, establish who those clients are, which will eventually use the proposed solution to be developed.

As a hypothesis of the problem, it is difficult for people with Parkinson's disease to travel to perform their physical rehabilitation therapies in health institutions.

The client's hypothesis is that they are people over 60 years of age who suffer from Parkinson's disease and are already undergoing physical rehabilitation treatment.

Both hypotheses will be validated from a survey of patients with Parkinson's disease to corroborate, or where appropriate, modify what is considered as a problem and client.

2.3   Validation of the Problem Hypothesis and the Client

To validate the hypotheses of the problem and the client previously formulated, a survey was applied, through a questionnaire, this in accordance with the restrictions presented by the COVID-19 pandemic. It should be noted that this questionnaire was carried out through an online tool and that it was applied to patients with Parkinson's disease that could be found through relatives and acquaintances who participated in the project.

As considerations of the questionnaire, it is specified that the responses are collected for scientific purposes only and they will be handled with the highest degree of privacy. At the time of the people responding, they were told not to provide personal data to comply with the aforementioned.

The computer tool for the application of the questionnaires was Google Questionnaires (https://docs.google.com/forms/d/e/1FAIpQLSdRsHYCwPDL3SkMIjV-BkNQtrjeXwo8FpJ7epjREzNhUm89xw/viewform), since it is easy to implement for the creation of a friendly interface with people when answering questions.

The questions that make up the questionnaire are shown in the following table (Table 1):

Table 1. Questionnaire to validate problem and customer hypotheses.

No	Questions
1	Gender:
2	Age:
3	How long have you been with treatment?
4	What is your treatment based on? a) Drugs b) Rehabilitation - Therapy c) Others (specify the patient)
5	Do you consider that your treatment has impacted on your economy?
6	What daily activities do you consider to be difficult to carry out? a) Basic Activities • Bath • Get dressed • Use the toilet • Eat • Get out of bed • Other (specify) b) Activities implemented: • Cook • Carry out household chores • Buy groceries • Taking medications • Traveling only by public transport • Laundry • Make phone calls • Other (specific)
7	During the development of the activities mentioned above, which of the following symptoms are the most recurrent? (You can select more than one) a) Tremors (upper limbs) b) Tremors (lower limbs) c) Muscle stiffness (upper limbs) d) Rigidity (lower limbs) e) Slow movement (bradykinesia) f) Balance problem g) Difficulty writing h) Other (specify)

(*continued*)

Table 1. (*continued*)

No	Questions
8	Of the following symptoms, which one would be the first to fix in the short term? a) Tremors (upper limbs) b) Tremors (lower limbs) c) Muscle stiffness (upper limbs) d) Rigidity (lower limbs) e) Slow movement (bradykinesia) f) Balance problem g) Difficulty writing h) Other (specify)
9	Do you do any physical therapy activities related to your illness? (If the answer is "Yes", go to question 9.1) So b) No 9.1. If the answer to question 9 was "Yes", describe what physical therapy you do
10	Do you currently use any medical equipment to help you with your rehabilitation therapy? Example: wheelchair, special spoons, walking sticks, among others. (If the answer is "Yes", go to question 10.1) 10.1. If the answer to question 10 was "Yes", write what medical equipment you use
11	What is the main difficulty/annoyance you face in your therapy?
12	At home, do exercises help you with your treatment? (If the answer is "Yes", go to question 12.1) 12.1. If the answer to question 12 was "Yes", write what exercises you do
13	Do you think that making use of medical equipment for your therapy at home makes your exercises easier?
14	What savings would you value most? on time b) Money c) Effort
15	What do you think would make therapy more accessible to you?

Some of the results obtained were:

In relation to Fig. 3, it is observed that 44% of those surveyed undergo rehabilitation therapy as treatment, which validates those patients carry out physical rehabilitation therapy activities for their Parkinson's disease.

In relation to Fig. 4, it is observed that the most recurrent symptoms are among tremors (upper limbs), balance problems, and slow movement (bradykinesia), which hinders their daily life, and of course that their transfer to medical appointments to carry out their physical rehabilitation therapies.

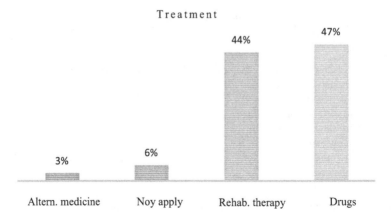

Fig. 3. Treatment carried out by the surveyed patients

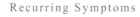

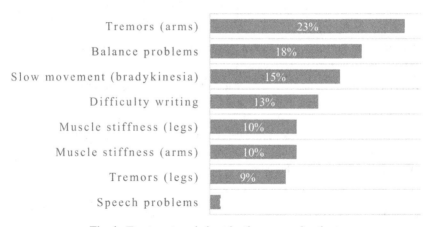

Fig. 4. Treatment carried out by the surveyed patients

Regarding the client's hypothesis, as can be seen in Fig. 5, it is observed that, in fact, patients over 60 years of age are mostly those who attend physical rehabilitation therapies, and that there is no distinction regarding gender.

2.4   Formulation of the Solution Hypothesis

Based on the detected needs of patients with Parkinson's disease, Fig. 3, it is established to think about devising a therapy proposal that they can carry out remotely and avoid going to their doctor's appointments. Beyond the fact of having to be transported, there is the fact of recurrent symptoms, where it takes a greater relevance to perform your rehabilitation physical therapy in the best way.

Ages of respondents

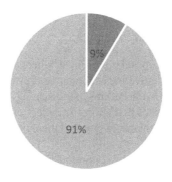

■ under 60 years   ■ over 60 years old

Fig. 5. Ages of the respondents patients

That is why the following solution hypothesis is established: having a technological platform that has electronic devices that allows to monitor the movements of patients remotely to perform a rehabilitation teletherapy.

To validate this solution hypothesis, the lean startup methodology [6] proposes to build a functional prototype that complies with the characteristics that allow to eliminate the detected need. The next step is to build a conceptual prototype so that customers can interact with it at a later stage.

There are symptoms related to Parkinson's disease, such as gait. Table 2 [7] shows the gait measures to take into account for a rehabilitation process; these same measures could be remotely monitored in order to provide adequate assistance when patients are executing it [8].

Table 2. Gait measures to monitor.

Disorders	Gait measures to monitor
Post-stroke	Gait velocity, time-distance measures, joint angles
Anterior cruciate ligament injury	Knee flexion, hip abduction-adduction
Knee replacement	Joint angle at different gait events, ground force reaction
Lower limb osteoarthritis	Gait speed, knee joint angle, hip angle, peak moments of knee extension, hip flexion and ankle plantar-flexion
Spinal cord injury	Gait speed, cadence, stride length
Prosthetics	Range of motion, energy storing, energy cost
Orthoses	Ankle joint angle, stride length

So a prototype platform that measures the march will be built, in order to offer remote guidance and assistance.

2.5 Construction of the Solution Prototype

A practical application of this proposal is presented, where a prototype of a technological platform that allows the quantitative measurement and evaluation of a remote rehabilitation program in individuals with Parkinson's disease is shown. It should be noted that this platform will have devices that allow the collection and analysis of precise and detailed information on the movements of physical therapies in patients with Parkinson's disease.

The proposed prototype consists of continuously monitoring the angles formed by the elbows, shoulders, arms, hips and knees; as well as the number of steps and the postural inclination of an individual with a diagnosis of Parkinson's disease who is under a certain physical rehabilitation therapy.

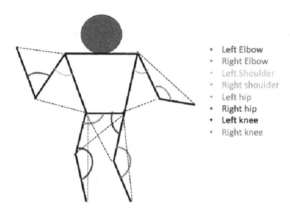

Fig. 6. Identification of angles for continuous monitoring during physical rehabilitation therapy

Figure 6 illustrates the identification and nomenclature of the angles used in continuous monitoring. For the identification and monitoring in real time of these angles, a 5 megapixel resolution video camera was used connected to a Google coral TPU development board [9], allows the use of BlazePose that is a convolutional neural network for high-fidelity body pose tracking, capable to infer 33 3D landmarks on the whole body from RGB video [10], including the shoulders, wrists, elbows, hips, knees and ankles.

3 Results

Figure 7 shows a volunteer subject making repeated movements from left to right, starting from a central position, in order to evaluate the magnitude of the movement of her head and shoulders. In Fig. 7.B are depicted the specific landmarks considered to extract the angles of movement that are graphed in Fig. 7.C.

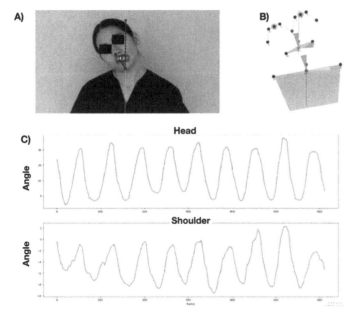

Fig. 7. Head and shoulder movements computed by the proposed system.

Figure 8 shows a volunteer subject with hands on waist, making repeated lateral flexions of trunk. Principal landmarks of mouth, shoulders, back tilt, pelvic tilt, flexion of the left and right elbows were considered to graph their respective angles.

Figure 9 shows a volunteer subject making repeated movements of her right hand touching her left shoulder, starting with the hands at the sides. Principal landmarks for elbows and shoulders were considered to graph their respective angles.

4   Discussions

A proposal was presented for the identification of business ideas in medical devices, highlighting in the first instance the formulation of hypotheses for the problem and the customer to be analyzed. These formulations were validated with surveys of patients with Parkinson's disease. Then a solution hypothesis was formulated that led to the construction of a conceptual functional prototype, which will soon also be validated with the patients.

Regarding the functional prototype, the technological components that make it up are very relevant, that is, those that make up the platform for the realization of physical rehabilitation teletherapy, which will allow monitoring the movements of patients with Parkinson's, in order to influence in the performance of their movements.

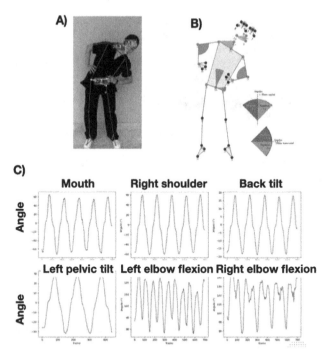

Fig. 8. Movements computed by the proposed system when the subject make repeated lateral flexions of trunk

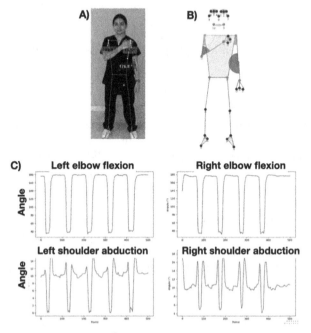

Fig. 9. Movements computed by the proposed system when the subject make repeated contralateral movements of her arms

5   Conclusions

A telerehabilitation prototype for the monitoring of postural disorders in patients with Parkinson's disease proposal was presented. This prototype was based on a methodology por the identification of business ideas in medical devices, highlighting in the first instance the formulation of hypotheses for the problem and the customer to be analyzed. These formulations were validated with surveys of patients with Parkinson's disease. Then a solution hypothesis was formulated that led to the construction of a conceptual functional prototype, which will soon also be validated with the patients.

As is known, gait analysis is usually carried out using subjective and qualitative approaches, such as human observation by the doctor and the opinion of the patient. Therefore, the main quantitative measures that can be derived are cadence, gait speed and distance traveled.

This rehabilitation prototype will provide a platform that will perform and interpret the measurements of the movements of the patients in a quantitative way, thus avoiding the misinterpretations derived from the observation of the doctors, and the opinion of the patients when they are consulted.

Regarding the functional prototype, the technological components that make it up are very relevant, that is, those that make up the platform for the realization of physical rehabilitation teletherapy, which will allow monitoring the movements of patients with Parkinson's, to influence in the performance of their movements.

The information shown in the results makes it possible to identify that it is possible to perform remote measurements in patients with Parkinson's in order to control and improve their movements.

Finally, discussions on the adoption of portable sensors for clinical measurements are being expanded through the review of case studies. The greater the use of these measurement instruments based on technological platforms by doctors and by patients themselves, the appropriate implementation within clinical practice may be required, in this case for patients with Parkinson's disease.

Acknowledgments. To the program UNAM-DGAPA-PAPIIT Project TA100921 Motor Telerehabilitation Platform for Parkinson's Disease.

References

1. Saracco, R.: Post-pandemic Scenarios – XIV – Telehealth. https://cmte.ieee.org/futuredirect ions/2021/04/16/post-pandemic-scenarios-xiv/. Accessed 10 July 2021
2. Raiano, L., Di Pino, G., Di Biase, L, Tombini, M., Tagliamonte, N.L., Formica, D.: PDMeter: a wrist wereable device for an at-home assessment of the Parkinson's disease rigidity. IEEE Trans. Neural Syst. Rehabil. Eng. **28**(6), 1325–1333 (2020). https://doi.org/10.1109/TNSRE. 2020.2987020
3. S., F. La industria de dispositivos médicos en México. https://www.expomed.com.mx/es/ conferencias/blog/contenido-dispositivos-medicos/la-industria-de-dispositivos-medicos-en-mexico.html. Accessed 10 July 2021

4. Valencia-Juliao, H.: Panorama del emprendimiento de base tecnológica en la salud. http://www.cienciamx.com/index.php/sociedad/politica-cientifica/16251-panorama-emprendimiento-base-tecnologica-salud. Accessed 10 July 2021

5. Hart, J.: The Art of the Storyboard: A Filmmaker's Introduction. https://books.google.nl/books?id=3WfmPt0gbagC&hl=es. Accessed 10 July 2021

6. Llamas-Fernández, F.J., Fernández-Rodríguez, J.C.: La metodología Lean Startup: desarrollo y aplicación para el emprendimiento. https://doi.org/10.21158/01208160.n84.2018. 1918. Accessed 10 July 2021

7. Chen, S., Lach, J., Lo, B., Yang, G.Z.: Towards pervasive gait analysis with wearable sensors: a systematic review. J. Biomed. Health Inform. **14**(8), 1521–1537 (2016). https://doi.org/10.1109/JBHI.2016.2608720

8. Chen, Y., Shen, C., Wei, X.S., Liu, L., Yang, J.: Adversarial posenet: a structure-aware convolutional network for human pose estimation. In: Proceedings of the IEEE International Conference on Computer Vision, pp. 1212–1221 (2017)

9. Cass, S.: Taking AI to the edge: Google's TPU now comes in a maker-friendly package. IEEE Spectr. **56**(5), 16–17 (2019)

10. Bazarevsky, V., et al.: BlazePose: on-device real-time body pose tracking. arXiv preprint arXiv:2006.10204 (2020)

Analysis of Medical Tourism and the Effect of Using Digital Tools to Profile Travelers in Mexico

Edmundo Arrioja-Castrejón$^{(\boxtimes)}$ 🆔 and Andrée Marie López-Fernández 🆔

Escuela de Ciencias Económicas y Empresariales, Universidad Panamericana, Augusto Rodin 498, Insurgentes Mixcoac, Benito Juárez, 03920 Ciudad de México, Mexico
earrioja@up.edu.mx

Abstract. The increase of internet services and the availability of new cutting-edge technology, as well as the use of mobile apps and devices, set a major challenge for medical tourism service providers. E-commerce sites and social networks are an important source for consumers' awareness and knowledge regarding the medical tourism business model in México which has grown at accelerated rates in recent years; therefore their use should be enhanced by formalizing this activity, and creating integrated commercial strategies [1].

Word-of-mouth and the Internet are consumers' preferred sources of information for medical tourism [2], where trust is elemental for the perception of quality online information [3]. The use of social networks as a means of reference and information based on other users' experiences and recommendations, as well as the use of mobile applications, have contributed to making electronic commerce increasingly profitable for companies that incorporate them in their business model.

This research analyzes the preferences of consumption of medical tourism services in Mexico to determine the effect of formalizing the offer of services with the help of a digital platform on the consumers' experiences.

The study seeks to determine, through the integration of different cluster methodologies, which are the profiles of medical tourism travelers to better predict their consumption habits and channel the various options available through the use of digital tools and social networks to promote the most attractive alternatives for consumers' benefit, which translates into higher sales impacting the entire value chain of this sector.

Keywords: Medical tourism · Digital platforms · Traveler profile · Consumer behavior

1 Introduction

Improving the experience of medical tourism consumers represents a major challenge for service providers in this sector, especially when considering consumer preferences and habits, ensuring confidentiality, safety, budget, promotions, and integrated packages

© ICST Institute for Computer Sciences, Social Informatics and Telecommunications Engineering 2021
Published by Springer Nature Switzerland AG 2021. All Rights Reserved
J. A. Marmolejo-Saucedo et al. (Eds.): COMPSE 2021, LNICST 393, pp. 143–161, 2021.
https://doi.org/10.1007/978-3-030-87495-7_10

that are currently available, with the use of Artificial Intelligence (AI) tools and routines to contemplate other alternatives that the customer has available according to their integrated profile as a patient and traveler.

This research analyzes the consumption habits and preferences of medical tourism services in Mexico to determine the effect on customer experience when formalizing the offer of services with the help of a digital platform. The overall objective of this research was to examine the consumer preferences of the medical tourism industry in Mexico and the impact of digital tools on their choice of a service provider.

The lack of use of digital tools, transparency and promotion in the medical tourism industry in Mexico, and its possible effects, led to the formulation of the following hypotheses: an increase in the transparency of medical tourism services in Mexico through the use of digital tools, has an effect on consumer purchase decision-making; and, the greater use of digital tools to make more information available about medical tourism, the greater the patient's willingness to consume services in Mexico.

1.1 Theoretical Framework

Considering the needs and preferences of medical tourism consumers using various tools to approach the relationship among consumers and service providers should be a priority [4]; the latter should occur while still contemplating additional factors, such as supporting the patient throughout their treatment and their companions to remain in a comfortable environment throughout their stay, and providing activities to make their trip more pleasant.

Medical Tourism

Tourism is a strategic activity for Mexico and contributes 8.4% to the national Gross Domestic Product (GDP). The hotel sector in Mexico represents the main source of income of this industry and is the source of work for millions of Mexican families who directly or indirectly depend on this activity [5].

Medical services in Mexico represent another important source of direct employment and social welfare by integrating many specialized professionals such as doctors, paramedics, and nurses, as well as other related service providers, such as scientists, administrators, assistants, stretcher-bearers, among many others. According to ProMexico's data for 2011 [6], private health institutions totaled nearly 13,500 practices (of which 62% were a specialty) and 34,807 beds.

According to ProMexico's 2013 health tourism report [6], the proportion of medical specialists among general doctors in Mexico is 63.4% above the average of the countries of the Organization for Economic Cooperation and Development (OECD); therefore, this sector represents a large source of income for many medical specialists and is an important generator of indirect jobs through its supply chain.

The private health sector has the greatest probability of benefiting from medical tourism in Mexico since it has been the only provider of medical tourism services, until now, relying solely on the support of local and federal governments [7].

The medical tourism industry in Mexico has had significant growth over the last few years until 2020. According to data obtained from Euromonitor International [8], as shown in Fig. 1 below, Mexico maintained sustained growth except for the years 2009, 2015, and 2016.

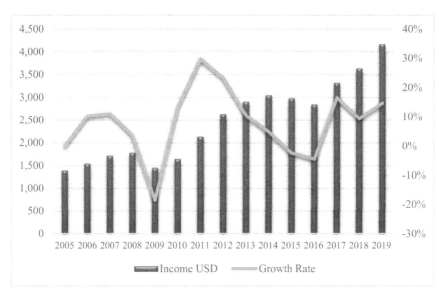

Fig. 1. Medical tourism revenue in Mexico in millions of dollars and annual growth rate.

In the period from 2005 to 2019, service providers and consumers, mainly in the United States and Canada, saw in Mexico an alternative to treat the 21 types of medical conditions (see Table 1) that can be programmed for care in clinics and hospitals, reaching growth figures close to 30% in just 2011 [9].

This is mainly due to the differential in price and the quality of the facilities and medical care that the country possesses. Mexico, together with Israel and Thailand, is one of Canada's preferred destinations for medical conditions (such as vision problems, dental implants, and gastric and aesthetic treatments) with sustained growth for Canadian consumers between 2013 and 2018 [10].

Medical tourism revenues in Mexico, according to 2018 data provided by the National Institute of Statistics and Geography (INEGI) [11], hovered around 7.1% of total revenue from international tourism, equivalent to approximately $1.6 billion dollars. If national foreign medical tourism is also considered, the figure increases in 2018 to more than $3,637 million and, at the end of 2019, to more than $4.175 million [8].

The North American market is an unbeatable opportunity for medical tourism in Mexico [10] due to proximity and prices of medical treatments in the United States and Canada. If the political and economic conditions of the country allow, it will be an important source of jobs, social welfare, and growth for many Mexicans looking for new opportunities because of the number of businesses and supply chains involved in these sectors. These conditions may only be given when medical tourism services are technically provided with the use of digital tools to bring the supply and demand of these services into contact [9].

Table 1. Major countries and medical tourism treatments in the world, data from the Medical Tourism Association – August 2020 (Figures in US dollars).

Treatment / Country	Colombia	Costa Rica	India	Israel	Jordan	Malaysia	Mexico	Poland	Singapore	Thailand	Turkey	USA
Angioplasty	7,100	13,800	5,700	7,500	5,000	8,000	10,400	5,300	13,400	4,200	4,800	28,200
Heart Bypass	14,800	27,000	7,900	28,000	14,400	12,100	27,000	14,000	17,200	15,000	13,900	123,000
Valve Replacement	10,450	30,000	9,500	28,500	14,400	13,500	28,200	19,000	16,900	17,200	17,200	170,000
Hip Replacement	8,400	13,600	7,200	36,000	8,000	8,000	13,500	5,500	13,900	17,000	13,900	40,364
Hip Resurfacing	10,500	13,200	9,700	20,100	9,000	12,500	12,500	9,200	16,350	13,500	10,100	28,000
Knee Replacement	7,200	12,500	6,600	25,000	9,500	7,700	12,900	8,200	16,000	14,000	10,400	35,000
Spinal Fusion	14,500	15,700	10,300	33,500	10,000	6,000	15,400	6,200	12,800	9,500	16,800	110,000
Dental Implant	1,200	800	900	1,200	1,000	1,500	900	925	2,700	1,720	1,100	2,500
Lap Band	8,500	9,450	7,300	17,300	7,000	8,150	6,500	6,700	9,200	11,500	8,600	14,000
Gastric Sleeve	11,200	11,500	7,300	20,000	7,500	8,400	8,900	9,400	11,500	9,900	12,900	16,500
Gastric Bypass	12,200	12,900	7,000	24,000	7,500	9,900	11,500	9,750	13,700	16,800	13,800	25,000
Hysterectomy	2,900	6,900	3,200	14,500	6,600	4,200	4,500	2,200	10,400	3,650	7,000	15,400
Breast Implants	2,500	3,500	3,000	3,800	4,000	3,800	4,500	3,900	8,400	3,500	4,500	6,400
Rhinoplasty	4,500	3,800	2,400	4,600	2,900	2,200	3,800	2,500	2,200	3,300	3,100	6,500
Face Lift	4,000	4,500	3,500	6,800	3,950	3,550	4,900	4,000	440	3,950	6,700	11,000
Liposuction	2,500	2,800	2,800	2,500	1,400	2,500	3,000	1,800	2,900	2,500	3,000	5,500
Tummy Tuck	3,500	5,000	3,500	10,900	4,200	3,900	4,500	3,550	4,650	5,300	4,000	8,000
Lasik (both eyes)	2,400	2,400	1,000	3,800	4,900	3,450	1,900	1,850	3,800	2,310	1,700	4,000
Cornea (per eye)	ND	9,800	2,800	ND	5,000	ND	ND	ND	9,000	3,600	7,000	17,500
Cataract surgery	1,600	1,700	1,500	3,700	2,400	3,000	2,100	750	3,250	1,800	1,600	3,500
IVF Treatment	5,450	ND	2,500	5,500	5,000	6,900	5,000	4,900	14,900	4,100	5,200	12,400

The Covid-19 pandemic during 2020 and 2021 has boosted the technification of many previously only face-to-face services and has accelerated the adoption of digital solutions and tools by companies and professionals [12].

It has been identified that the most widely used media by the offer of medical services are the Internet with 26%, radio and television with 14% each, the yellow pages directories with 12% and, finally, newspapers and magazines with 10% each [13].

Digital Tools

The literature review highlights the need for digital tools based on Artificial Intelligence (AI) for the analysis of human behavior in the fields of understanding, perception, problem-solving and decision-making to reproduce them with the help of a computer [14].

AI is a concept that has been studied for several decades but has been enhanced mainly in recent years because of the number of applications and the impact it is having on modern society, as well as the consequences of this technology on people's behavior and decision-making [15]. However, projects that integrate technology should focus more on information and less on technology [16], as the goal of any system is to provide information or execute a data-based action.

Big Data

Multiple companies are investing large amounts of resources in information technologies and data experts to extract valuable information from the large volumes of data available on networks. Those companies and individuals who respond more efficiently and recognize that competing in the world of analytics will provide them with greater competitive advantages will be the main beneficiaries of this technological revolution [17].

Information may come from social networks, images, and sensors on devices, among many other sources and, because of this, all service providers must base decision-making on evidence and data. Organizations also need to process and identify patterns in very large datasets and translate them into useful business information [18].

The use of data is very important, particularly in regards to the exploitation given to them through advanced analytics for the personal care industry [19], which is closely related to some treatments sought-after under the model of medical tourism such as dental and breast implants, gastric bypass and liposuction. A study on healthcare application showcases a variety of data sources, their constant interrelationship, and the applications available for processing and leveraging personal care [20].

There are several key elements to consider in handling large volumes of data: veracity, variability or complexity, and value [21]. Therefore, to the extent that data is classified through the use of technology, service providers such as hospitals, clinics, airlines, hotels, and restaurants, all of them related to medical tourism, will be able to have information available in real-time to boost their business; thus, they will be able to offer goods and services focused on customers with a greater degree of acceptance.

Currently, internet marketing and social media companies use their members' large volumes of data to analyze them for commercial gain, which is particularly "evidenced by the burgeoning popularity of many social networks such as Twitter, Facebook, and LinkedIn" [22].

Social Networks and Mobility

Social media and the internet have helped to obtain simultaneous, real-time information, and segment different types of consumers by their interests, education, sex, location, and marital status [23]. This helps companies like Amazon, Google, and Facebook anticipate people's needs and consumption habits so they can produce and deliver products and services closer to everyone's preferences.

The use of mobile devices has intensified the use of the internet for multiple personal applications which provide a means to develop programs capable of distinguishing locations and displacements; they also allow the location of consumers at all times and determine their mobility and consumption habits, which helps companies offer real-time services to customers approaching the provider's location [24]. The availability of mobile devices and the COVID-19 pandemic effect is revolutionizing the use of such technologies globally.

A study on group recommender systems describes a social media-based approach to referral systems for the tourism industry, where a group profile is built analyzing not only user preferences but also social relationships between members of the whole group [25]. This is highly useful if we consider groups with common health problems such as cornea disease or heart valve transplants.

Regarding social media, consumers' trust positively impacts brand assessment and their emotional response to advertisement [26]. As such, websites and social media are important platforms for healthcare provides as well as medical tourists to both search for and provide information on experiences, services, destinations, firms, costs, amongst others [27]. Therefore, data and information retrieved online, and particularly social media, have a significant impact on medical tourism consumers' decision-making.

Recommendation Systems

Recommendation systems have been developed in parallel with the Internet, initially built with demographic filters, based on content [28]; and, these systems are currently incorporating social media information and using device data through the Internet of Things (IoT).

A study which examined the landscape of hybrid recommendation systems introduced a system that combines knowledge-based recommendations and collaborative filters to suggest restaurants [29], could be the basis for the development and optimization of a system like this useful for medical tourism since they are services with common characteristics.

There are important achievements in the tourism industry that have been particularly benefited by the new technological advances that arise day by day. For instance, a study showed the development of an Artificial Intelligence (AI) software agent, called Traveler, which helps users select their trip [30]. This solution combines collaboration methods with content-based recommendations and demographic data about customers to suggest tailor-made vacation packages. It is important to analyze this development in greater depth to determine whether it is possible to adapt it to consider all the categories and subcategories that have arisen from interviews and future medical tourism consumer surveys.

Artificial Intelligence analytical-based recommendation systems and advanced routines for determining customer behavior in tourism are a phenomenon of increasing relevance to the economic impact it represents for AI companies. As such, it is important to study the role played by information technologies in the competitiveness of the service providers [31].

2 Methodology

The objective of this research is to segment the population of medical tourists and understand their profile. We worked with mixed data using a special metric (Gower distance) to achieve better results. This document analyzes data from international medical tourism associations: Patients Beyond Borders and Medical Tourism Association. It also analyzes data from specialized reports from Euromonitor International in August 2020 and other data sources detailed below.

2.1 Cluster Segmentation Analysis

Clustering segmentation refers to a broad set of techniques for finding groups, or subgroups, within a data set. When we carry out this grouping, we seek to divide the observations so that those belonging to the same group are quite like each other, while those belonging to other groups are different.

The model used in this study began with a correlation analysis to determine if the variables have a significant relationship. Subsequently, a cluster segmentation analysis for mixed data was performed using hierarchical agglomerative, k-means, and k-medoids to identify the relationship between the study's variables and the groups of traveler profiles, considering the sample under study and the effect of the selection of reservation tools on those profiles.

The objective of comparing a series of methodologies is to be able to select an ideal methodology for the treatment of the analyzed data. The following steps were considered in the development of the segmentation model:

1. Validation of variable correlation and trends in clustering using Hopkins statistic
2. Selection of the number of partitions to be made
3. Selection of the best cluster segmentation algorithm using Dunn index
4. Validation of the generated clusters using Silhouette coefficient.

Hierarchical Agglomerative

Hierarchical agglomerative grouping classifies objects into groups according to their similarity and, through a repetitive process, pairs of groups are successively merged until all groups merge into one large group containing all objects [32].

Clustering by K-means

Clustering by K-means is an effective algorithm to divide a data set into K groups according to the similarity of the observations [33].

Let X1,..., Xn a sample of observations. Where a partition of K groups of observations is defined by C1,..., Ck, where $C1 \cup C1 \cup \cdots \cup Ck = \{X1, \ldots, Xn\}$ and $Ci \cap Cj = \emptyset; i \neq j$.

The objective is solving the minimization problem (Eq. 1).

$$\underset{C1, \ldots, Ck}{min} = \left\{ \sum_{k=1}^{k} W(Ck) \right\} \tag{1}$$

Where, W(Ck) is a measure of the intra-cluster variation Ck, which must solve the quadratic Euclidean distance (Eq. 2).

$$W(Ck) = \frac{1}{|Ck|} \sum_{i,i' \in Ck} \sum_{j=1}^{p} \left(Xij - Xi'j \right)^2 \tag{2}$$

Where |Ck| denotes the number of observations in cluster K, and X_{ij} is the value of observation i in variable j.

Clustering by K-medoids

K-medoids is a partition clustering technique where each cluster is represented by an element of the cluster, these are points known as the medoids. The term medoid refers to an object within a cluster for which the average dissimilarity between it and all other members of the cluster is minimal [33]. K-medoids is less sensitive to noise and outliers because it uses the medoids as cluster centers instead of the centroids (used in k-means).

The K-medoids algorithm is a robust alternative to K-means to partition a data set into groups. In the K-medoids method, each group is represented by a selected object within the cluster. The selected objects are called medoids and correspond to the most central points located within the cluster.

The PAM (Partitioning Around Medoids) algorithm is the most common grouping method [34], that requires that the user know the data and indicate the appropriate data and number of clusters to be produced.

Hopkins Statistic

For validation of randomness, we use the Hopkins statistic (Eq. 3) that tells us whether the study database behaves uniformly or not. This allows us to define if the data are subject to clustering. This statistic measures the probability that a given data set is generated by data of a uniform distribution [35].

$$H = \frac{\sum_{i=1}^{n} Y_i}{\sum_{i=1}^{n} X_i + \sum_{i=1}^{n} Y_i} \tag{3}$$

Where $X_i = dist(p_i, p_j)$ is the distance for each observation from its closest neighbor and $Y_i = dist(q, q_j)$ is the distance for each point from its closest neighbor in a data set simulated using a uniform distribution [36].

Gower Distance for Mixed Data

A popular option for clustering is to use the Euclidean distance. However, this metric is only valid for continuous variables. Thus, for a clustering algorithm to produce reasonable results, we must use a distance metric that can handle mixed data types such as those contemplated in this study [37]. Therefore, we will use the Gower distance (Eq. 4):

$$GOW_{jk} = \frac{\sum_{i=1}^{n} W_{ijk} S_{ijk}}{\sum_{i=1}^{n} W_{ijk}} \tag{4}$$

Where $W_{ijk} = 0$ if the objects j and k cannot be compared for the variable i if X_{ij} or X_{jk} are not known. Gower's distance concept indicates that for each type of variable, a particular measurement scale is used that works well for that type and scaled between 0 and 1. A linear join is then calculated using user-specified weights to create the final distance matrix [38].

Dunn Index

The Dunn index (Eq. 5) is an internal cluster validation measure that allows you to calculate the distance between each of the objects in the group and the objects in the other groups [39]. This index calculates the minimum of this pairwise distance as the separation between clusters (min.separation) and uses the maximum distance within the cluster as the intracluster compactness.

$$D = \frac{min.separation}{max.diameter} \tag{5}$$

Silhouette Coefficient

The Silhouette coefficient (Eq. 6) was used as an optimization criterion to determine the number of partitions in a cluster using a measure of the quality of the cluster classification [40].

$$Silhouette = \frac{1}{N} \sum_{i=1}^{N} \frac{d_i - s_i}{\max\{d_i - s_i\}} \tag{6}$$

2.2 Definition of Variables

Data were first obtained from the main medical treatments that are programmed under the medical tourism modality and from the main countries where they are marketed. Then a survey was carried out with a sample of 100 tourists and consumers of medical tourism incorporating some variables defined in a previous study carried out in Malaysia [41], with the purpose of identifying travel preferences to better establish the traveler profile.

From the questions asked, the following variables were obtained: type of trip (business, pleasure, or both), gender (male or female), age, number of trips made per year (1, 2, 3, 4, 5, 6, 7 or +), average expense per trip in Mexican Pesos, preferred type of transportation (air, land, or sea), preferred place of travel (between beach and city) and preferred reservation medium (internet/mobile app, social media or travel agency/phone). For this exercise, we considered a sample of 51 men and 49 women.

From that database, the selection variables were converted by assigning values 0 and 1 to convert them into dichotomic and trichotomic variables (see Table 2), and focus on determining which factors should be contemplated when designing a digital tool based on the user preferences; the latter resulted in the following variable relationship:

Table 2. Variables analyzed according to a sample of 100 medical tourists surveyed.

Variables		Data type	Description of variables
Expenditure		Weights figure	Average travel expense
Age		Figure in Years	Traveler's age
Travel		Whole number	Number of trips per year
Gender	1 – Male	Dichotomic	Gender (male or female)
	0 - Female	variable	
Type of Transport	Aerial	Trichotomic variable	Air mean preference
	Terrestrial		Land mean preference
	Maritime		Maritime mean preference
Place	1 – City	Dichotomic	Travel place preference (city or beach)
	0 - Beach	variable	
Type of Trip	Business	Trichotomic variable	Higher business travel frequency
	Pleasure		Increased frequency of pleasure travel
	Both		Mixed travel frequency
Reservation medium	Internet_App	Trichotomic variable	Online booking or App preference
	Social_Network		Social media booking preference
	Agency_Phone		Booking preference by agency / phone

3   Results

3.1   Correlation Analysis

From the above data, we can see that there are 3 variables associated with the reservation medium, 3 variables associated with the type of transport, 4 variables associated with the traveler profile, and 1 variable associated with the place. Considering a sample of 100 travelers of medical tourism, we use the correlation analysis to study the relationship between the set of variables associated with the traveler profile with the variables linked to the type of reservation and quantify the number of existing independent dimensions.

The variables associated with the traveler's profile are Expense, Age, Travel, and Gender. The variables linked to the reservation type are Internet_App, Social_Network, and Agency_Phone. In addition, the variable Gender is an indicator variable from 0 to 1, where 1 indicates the consumer is male and 0 indicates the consumer is female.

Table 3 below shows the descriptive analysis of the variables studied, where we can see that we have 3 quantitative (Expense, Travel, Age) and 7 qualitative variables (Gender, Air, Terrestrial, Maritime, Internet_App, Social_Network, Agency_Phone).

Below are the 3 sets of grouped variables used in this study, of which we will only use in this analysis the reservation group (reservation type, composed of the variables: Internet_App, Social_Network, and Agency_Phone), and traveler information (traveler's profile, consisting of the variables Expense, Travel, Age, Gender), to be able to determine if there is a correlation among these variables, and see if the use of digital tools such as the Internet, mobile applications or social networks have a significant relationship with the type of user profile. We can see that the correlations within and between the 2 selected sets of variables in the database are as follows (see Table 4):

Table 3. Descriptive analysis of variables, using data from 100 surveys conducted on medical tourism travelers in 2019

Descriptive	Expenditure	Travel	Age	Gender	Place	Air	Terrestrial	Maritime	Internet_App	Social_Network	Agency_Phone
Min.:	5362	1.00	20.00	0.00	0.00	0.00	0.00	0.00	0.00	0.00	0.00
1st Qu.:	24659	2.00	34.75	0.00	0.00	0.00	0.00	0.00	0.00	0.00	0.00
Mediate:	45471	4.00	45.00	1.00	1.00	1.00	0.00	0.00	1.00	0.00	0.00
Mean :	44022	3.82	46.87	0.51	0.55	0.60	0.33	0.07	0.55	0.17	0.28
3rd Qu.:	62596	6.00	62.25	1.00	1.00	1.00	1.00	0.00	1.00	0.00	1.00
Max.:	79857	7.00	75.00	1.00	1.00	1.00	1.00	1.00	1.00	1.00	1.00

Table 4. Correlation of variables, data from 100 surveys on medical tourism travelers in 2019

Correlation	Expense	Travel	Age	Gender	Internet_App	Social_Network	Agency_Phone
Expense	1.0000	0.0113	0.0302	-0.0200	0.1029	-0.0523	-0.0703
Travel	0.0113	1.0000	-0.0103	0.0214	0.3535	-0.0644	-0.3378
Age	0.0302	-0.0103	1.0000	-0.1026	-0.0270	-0.3616	0.3324
Gender	-0.0200	0.0214	-0.1026	1.0000	-0.0020	0.1241	-0.1016
Internet_App	0.1029	0.3535	-0.0270	-0.0020	1.0000	-0.5003	-0.6894
Social_Network	-0.0523	-0.0644	-0.3616	0.1241	-0.5003	1.0000	-0.2822
Agency_Phone	-0.0703	-0.3378	0.3324	-0.1016	-0.6894	-0.2822	1.0000

As we can see in Table 4, there is a clear correlation between the age and the type of reservation; this correlation is positive at older ages in relation to the telephone or travel agency reservation method, and negative in relation to the Internet and social networks. There is also a positive correlation between average expenses and travel frequency.

3.2 Hopkins Statistic and Gower Distances for Mixed Data

First, we can see that Hopkins statistic shows the probability that a given data set is generated by data of a uniform distribution, using R tool is: $H = 0.5006383$, this implies that the grouping to be identified is not random and that there is an underlying pattern.

Next, we see that Gower's distance can be calculated on a line using the daisy function in R. Note that due to a positive result in the variable enrolled, a record transformation is performed internally through the type of argument. Instructions for performing additional transformations, such as factors might be considered asymmetrical binaries (such as rare events).

As a sanity control, we can print the most similar (see Table 5) and different (see Table 6) pair in the data to see if it makes sense. In this case, the person aged 32, whose average expense is 36,835, and the person of age 31 whose average expense is 41,743, are the most similar given the 11 characteristics used in the distance calculation:

Table 5. Generating similar pairs of data using Gower distance

Expense	Travel	Age	Gender	Place	Air	Terrestrial	Maritime	Internet_App	Social_Network
36835	4	32	0	1	1	0	0	1	0
41743	4	31	0	1	1	0	0	1	0

While on the contrary, the person aged 71, whose average travel expense is 17,675 and the 22-year-old whose average spend is 75,504 are the most different:

Table 6. Generating different pairs of data using Gower distance

Expense	Travel	Age	Gender	Place	Air	Terrestrial	Maritime	Internet_App	Social_Network
17675	6	71	0	1	0	1	0	0	0
75504	1	22	1	0	0	0	1	0	1

3.3 Clustering Methods Comparison

Below is the comparative (see Table 7) of the 3 cluster segmentation methods proposed, where we can see that the hierarchical agglomerative model for 3 partitions is the one that reports the highest parameters using Dunn index; however, after applying the final validation using Silhouette coefficient, we can see that the difference between hierarchical agglomerative and K-medoids method is minimal, so we will select the K-medoids method for the final analysis as it is a less sensitive model to noise and outliers.

Table 7. Comparison of the proposed clustering segmentation methods

Clustering segmentation	Clusters:	2	3	4	5	6
Hierarchical	Connectivity	2.2151	8.2044	8.8405	9.4627	11.0516
	Dunn	0.445	0.5309	0.5552	0.6109	0.6109
	Silhouette	0.3591	0.3292	0.3679	0.4034	0.3949
K-means	Connectivity	4.5262	6.1825	8.8405	9.4627	11.0516
	Dunn	0.4525	0.4776	0.5552	0.6109	0.6109
	Silhouette	0.3669	0.3444	0.3679	0.4034	0.3949
K-medoids (PAM)	Connectivity	5.9893	17.9833	28.2437	35.9425	29.8905
	Dunn	0.4525	0.3068	0.2028	0.2028	0.2028
	Silhouette	0.356	0.3268	0.3314	0.2725	0.3093

3.4   Cluster with Mixed Data Using K-medoids

For an algorithm yet to choose to group observations, we must first define some notion of (dis)similarity between observations.

There are a variety of metrics to help choose the number of clusters to extract in cluster analysis. We will use silhouette width, an internal validation metric that is an aggregate measure of how similar an observation is to a cluster compared to a nearest neighbor cluster. The metric can range from −1 to 1, where the highest values are better. After calculating the Silhouette width for clusters ranging from 2 to 10 for the PAM algorithm (which uses a partition around medoids), for the analyzed data, we can see in Fig. 2, that 3 clusters yield the highest initial value:

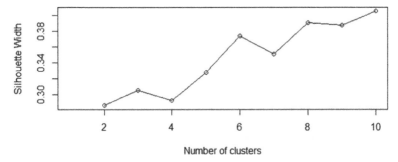

Fig. 2. Silhouette coefficient width chart to validate the number of clusters

One way to visualize many variables in a space of lower dimensions is with the graph t-SNE. This method is a dimension reduction technique that attempts to preserve the local structure to make clusters visible in a 2D or 3D plane (see Fig. 3). In this case, the graph shows the three well-separated clusters that PAM could detect:

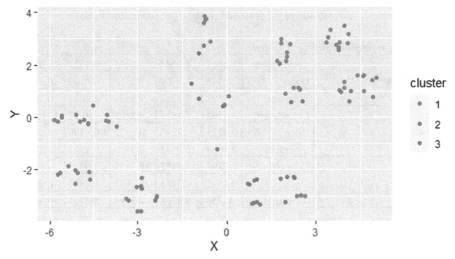

Fig. 3. Cluster scatter chart using the R tool with survey data conducted on medical tourism travelers in 2019

3.5   Cluster Validation Using Average Silhouette Width

The Silhouette width coefficient is used to validate the quality of the cluster and determine how well the observations were classified; higher values imply good classification (see Table 8), negative values mean badly classified observations and values of 0 mean that there is a possible overlap.

Table 8. Cluster widths using Silhouette coefficient

Cluster	Size	Average Silhouette width
1	41	0.42
2	34	0.3
3	25	0.21

To validate the number of clusters selected, we use the average Silhouette width. In Fig. 4 below, we can see the quality of the cluster created with K-medoids, in fact a Silhouette coefficient is generated for each observation, and the graph shows how

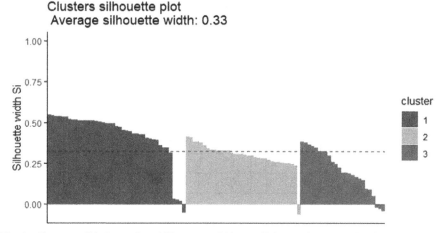

Fig. 4. Cluster validation using Silhouette width coefficient using R tool with survey data conducted on medical tourism travelers in 2019

many are correctly classified, how many can be overlaps and how many would be in the inappropriate cluster (the negative ones).

After running the algorithm and selecting 3 clusters, we can interpret the clusters by running a summary on each one, based on the following results:

Cluster 1 is mainly the profile of the Frequent/Air/Modern Traveler with average spending levels and frequent travel in the year, likes to book by electronic means and prefers to travel by plane, is the typical traveler who is looking for airlines and seeks comfort first.

Cluster 2, on the other hand, is mainly the profile of the Saver/Land/Modern Traveler with low spending levels and moderate travel in the year, that normally likes to book by electronic means and prefers to travel by land, and is the typical globetrotter.

Cluster 3 is mainly the profile of the Occasional/Air/Traditional Traveler, with the lowest levels of travel per year, average expenditure and that since it is not a frequent flyer prefers traditional means of reservation and the least possible complications.

Another benefit of the PAM algorithm, concerning interpretation, is that medoids serve as examples of each group (Table 9).

It is noteworthy that the male person, age 43 and average travel expense of 56,483, is the medoid of the Frequent/Air/Modern Traveler cluster, the male person, age 42 and average travel expense of 18,543, is the medoid of the Saving/Land/Modern Traveler cluster, and the female person, age 47 and average travel expense of 67,968, is the medoid of the Occasional/Air/Traditional Traveler cluster.

Table 9. Generation of medoids using the PAM algorithm

Cluster medoid	Expense	Travel	Age	Gender	Place	Air	Terrestrial	Maritime	Internet_App	Social_Network	Agency_Phone
1	56483	5	43	1	1	1	0	0	1	0	0
2	18543	6	42	1	1	0	1	0	1	0	0
3	67968	1	47	0	0	1	0	0	0	0	1

4   Conclusions

Consumers mostly travel from the United States, Canada and Western Europe to Asia and Latin America for medical tourism [42]. Common reasons may include insufficient insurance coverage, high costs of procedures [43] and/or even high deductibles. A study on medical tourism in Malaysia, found that demographics, such as age and sex, motivations, such as value for money, medical service quality and secondary services, as well as the type of procedure, were determining factors in the profile of medical tourists [41]. Another regarding medical tourism in India, found that it is common for medical tourists to incorporate travel plans during their medical procedure trip [44]. And, a study on expectation confirmation perspective suggested that consumer satisfaction is well associated with their expectation confirmation which may be derived from the actual performance of the medical service [45]. Thus, the study's findings are significantly related to results from previous studies in relation to medical tourism in other countries.

A key factor today to increase the competitiveness of medical tourism service providers is to take advantage of the exponential increase in internet purchases. The use of social networks as a means of reference and knowledge of recommendations based on other users' experiences, as well as the use of mobile applications have contributed to make e-commerce increasingly profitable for companies and those who incorporate it within their operating model. From the doctors who use social networks to advertise, the following social networks are identified as the most widely used: Facebook and YouTube with 32% each, Google with 18%, and Twitter and Pinterest with 9% each [13].

The use of digital tools to take advantage of the large volume of information that is on the Internet and social networks will give a competitive advantage to medical tourism service providers, especially considering new generations; as can be seen in the results, they prefer to interact with internet sites, social networks, e-commerce portals, whether through computers or mobile applications, than through a travel agency or a telephone advisor. Therefore, it is a significant opportunity to use recommendation systems based on Artificial Intelligence (AI) algorithms that can filter and channel consumers of these medical tourism services to the specialist, hospital, or clinic that can provide quality care, considering their budget, interests, and condition.

Based on the results obtained from the cluster segmentation analysis, we can conclude that consumers of medical tourism services in Mexico can be categorized into 3 different profiles based on their preferences and consumption habits, where the reservation method is a differentiating factor that is associated with the frequency of travel and the age of the participants within the sample analyzed in this research. Thus, results indicate that digital tools, in fact, positively influence consumer decision-making. Further, having clearly identified profiles of medical tourists will allow service providers to offer a better user experience focused on attention and improve contact conditions, which may increase patient's willingness to consume services in Mexico.

Therefore, we can also conclude according to the results obtained from the applied models that digital tools, such as the Internet, mobile applications, and social networks have a direct and positive effect on the behavior of consumers of medical tourism services in Mexico, which allow determining the type of profile of the traveler accurately, in addition to being increasingly used as a reservation method for the selection and contracting of these services, which confirms what is commented by several of the authors reviewed in the theoretical framework such as [13, 23, 25] and [12].

The study's main limitation is the sample, as results cannot be generalized. As a future line of research, it is contemplated to integrate the segmentation of the clusters into a platform for the data processing of medical tourists, as well as the generation of automatic reports that could be consulted automatically through the cloud.

References

1. Taufik, N.A., Sulistiadi, W.: The impact of medical tourism industry for the hospital services and marketing activities: a systematic review. J. Adm. Rumah Sakit **5**(1), 42–48 (2018)
2. Lam, C.C.C., Du Cros, H., Vong, T.N.L.: Macao's potential for developing regional Chinese medical tourism. Tour. Rev. **66**, 68–82 (2011)
3. Moslehifar, M.A., Ibrahim, N.A., Sandaran, S.C.: Assessing the quality of trust features on website content of top hospitals for medical tourism consumers. J. Komun. Malays. J. Commun. **32**(1), 469–489 (2016)
4. Kim, S., Arcodia, C., Kim, I.: Critical success factors of medical tourism: the case of South Korea. Int. J. Environ. Res. Public Health **16**(24), 4964 (2019)
5. Secretaria de Turismo: El gran motor de la economía nacional (2018)
6. ProMéxico: Turismo de Salud. Tur. Salud, pp. 1–2 (2013)
7. Orozco Núñez, E., et al.: An overview of Mexico's medical tourism industry – the cases of Mexico City and Monterrey (2014)
8. Euromonitor International: Medical Tourism Report (2020)
9. Euromonitor International: Global medical tourism briefing: a fast growing niche market (2011)
10. Becker, S.: Opportunities and caveats of medical tourism in Canada (2014)
11. INEGI: Encuesta de Turismo de Internación (2018)
12. Garcia-Muñoz, C., Pérez Sánchez, B., Navarrete Torres, M.: Las empresas ante el COVID-19. Rev. Investig. Gest. Ind. Ambient. Segur. salud en el Trab. GISST **2934**, 85–101 (2020)
13. Montiel, J.: Estrategias publicitarias en línea utilizadas por la oferta de turismo médico plástico y estético: el caso de Tijuana, Baja California, México. Online advertising strategies used by the supply of plastic and aesthetic medical tourism: Case study of T. Int. J. Mark. Commun. New Media **3**(June), 106–117 (2015)

14. Hardy, T.: (IA: inteligencia artificial). Polis Rev. la Univ. Boliv. **1**(2), 23 (2001)
15. Dwivedi, Y.K., et al.: Artificial intelligence (AI): multidisciplinary perspectives on emerging challenges, opportunities, and agenda for research, practice and policy. Int. J. Inf. Manage. (2019)
16. Marchand, D.A., Peppard, J.: Why IT fumbles analytics: tech projects should focus less on technology and more on information. Harv. Bus. Rev. (January-February 2013), 104–112 (2013)
17. Davenport, T.H., Patil, D.J.: Data scientist: the sexiest job of the 21st century. Harv. Bus. Rev. (October 2012), 70–76 (2012)
18. McAfee, A., Brynjolfsson, E.: Big data: the management revolution. Harv. Bus. Rev. (October 2012), 60–68 (2012)
19. Raghupathi, W., Raghupathi, V.: Big data analytics in healthcare: promise and potential. Heal. Inf. Sci. Syst. **2**, 1–10 (2014)
20. Koh, H.C., Tan, G.: Data mining applications in healthcare. J. Healthc. Inf. Manag. **19**(2), 64–72 (2011)
21. Gandomi, A., Haider, M.: Beyond the hype: big data concepts, methods, and analytics. Int. J. Inf. Manage. **35**(2), 137–144 (2015)
22. Aggarwal, C.C.: An introduction to social network data analytics. In: Aggarwal, C. (ed.) Social Network Data Analytics, pp. 1–15. Springer, Boston (2011). https://doi.org/10.1007/978-1-4419-8462-3_1
23. Angulo Toro, L.S.: Big data y neuromarketing como herramientas útiles para medir el comportamiento del consumidor en la industria de telecomunicaciones con el fin de crear con mayor precisión. Universidad Católica de Santiago de Guayaquil (2019)
24. Naveed, M.: Online learning based contextual model for mobility prediction BT - evolving ambient intelligence. In: O'Grady, M.J., et al. (eds.) Evolving Ambient Intelligence. AmI 2013. Communications in Computer and Information Science, vol. 413, pp. 313–319. Springer, Cham (2013). https://doi.org/10.1007/978-3-319-04406-4_32
25. Christensen, I., Schiaffino, S., Armentano, M.: Social group recommendation in the tourism domain. J. Intell. Inform. Syst. **47**(2), 209–231 (2016). https://doi.org/10.1007/s10844-016-0400-0
26. Hahn, I., Scherer, F., Basso, K., Santos, M.: Consumer trust in and emotional response to advertisements on social media and their influence on brand evaluation. Braz. Bus. Rev. **13**(4), 49–71 (2016)
27. Medhekar, A.: The role of social media for knowledge dissemination in medical tourism. In: Medical Tourism, pp. 132–161 (2017)
28. Bobadilla, J., Ortega, F., Hernando, A., Gutiérrez, A.: Recommender systems survey. Knowl.-Based Syst. **46**, 109–132 (2013)
29. Burke, R.: Hybrid recommender systems: Survey and experiments. User Model. User-Adapted Interact. **12**(4), 331–370 (2002)
30. Schiaffino, S., Amandi, A.: Building an expert travel agent as a software agent. Expert Syst. Appl. **36**(2 PART 1), 1291–1299 (2009)
31. Martínez, J., Majó, J., Casadesús, M.: El uso de las tecnologías de la información en el sector hotelero. In: Turitec 2006: VI Congreso nacional turismo y tecnologías de la información y las comunicaciones, pp. 1–13 (2006)
32. Ward, J.H.: Hierarchical grouping to optimize an objective function. J. Am. Stat. Assoc. **58**(301), 236–244 (1963)
33. Loy-García, G., Rodríguez-Aguilar, R., Marmolejo-Saucedo, J.-A.: An analytical intelligence model to discontinue products in a transnational company. In: Vasant, P., Zelinka, I., Weber, G.-W. (eds.) ICO 2020. AISC, vol. 1324, pp. 812–822. Springer, Cham (2021). https://doi.org/10.1007/978-3-030-68154-8_70

34. Park, H.S., Jun, C.H.: A simple and fast algorithm for K-medoids clustering. Expert Syst. Appl. **36**(2 PART 2), 3336–3341 (2009)
35. Banerjee, A., Davé, R.N.: Validating clusters using the Hopkins statistic. In: IEEE International Conference on Fuzzy Systems, vol. 1, pp. 149–153 (2004)
36. Hopkins, B., Skellam, J.G.: A new method for determining the type of distribution of plant individuals. Ann. Bot. **18**(2), 213–227 (1954)
37. Tuerhong, G., Kim, S.B.: Gower distance-based multivariate control charts for a mixture of continuous and categorical variables. Expert Syst. Appl. **41**(4 PART 2), 1701–1707 (2014)
38. Gower, J.C.: A general coefficient of similarity and some of its properties. Biometrics **27**(4), 857 (1971)
39. Dunn, J.C.: A fuzzy relative of the ISODATA process and its use in detecting compact well-separated clusters. J. Cybern. **3**(3), 32–57 (1973)
40. Gentle, J.E., Kaufman, L., Rousseeuw, P.J.: Finding groups in data: an introduction to cluster analysis. Biometrics **47**(2), 788 (1991)
41. Musa, G., Thirumoorthi, T., Doshi, D.: Travel behaviour among inbound medical tourists in Kuala Lumpur. Curr. Issues Tour. **15**(6), 525–543 (2012)
42. Hopkins, L., Labonté, R., Runnels, V., Packer, C.: Medical tourism today: What is the state of existing knowledge. J. Public Health Policy **31**(2), 185–198 (2010)
43. Lew, A.A., Hall, C.M., Williams, A.M.: The Wiley Blackwell Companion to Tourism. Wiley, Oxford (2014)
44. Sajjad, R.: Edical tourism in India: an empirical analysis of the demographic profile and perception of medical tourists. MAGNT Res. Rep. **3**(8), 150–168 (2015)
45. Chou, S.Y., Kiser, A.I.T., Rodriguez, E.L.: An expectation confirmation perspective of medical tourism. J. Serv. Sci. Res. **4**(2), 299–318 (2012)

Performance Evaluation of Healthcare Systems Using Data Envelopment Analysis

Itzel Viridiana González-Badillo[✉] and Zaida Estefanía Alarcón-Bernal

Universidad Nacional Autónoma de México, Circuito Escolar 04360, C.U., Coyoacán, 04510 Mexico City, Mexico
itzel.gonzalez@ingenieria.unam.edu, zaida.alarcon@unam.mx

Abstract. This paper studies the context of 39 different countries' healthcare systems up to 2019 by applying the output-oriented variable return-to-scale model (VRS) of data envelopment analysis. 4 input variables (health expenditure per capita and beds, physicians, and nurses per thousand people) should result in the best 4 output results (life expectancy at birth, death rate per thousand people by communicable and non-communicable diseases, percentage of diabetes prevalence and mortality of cardiovascular diseases, cancer, diabetes or chronic respiratory disease). Efficient and super-efficient systems are identified and Mexico's system is discussed as an example.

Keywords: Linear programming · Health care logistics · Operations research

1 Introduction

It is widely and increasingly known that healthcare is an essential priority to any society. Thus, it is important to analyze and discuss how a healthcare system is performing in order to identify the most important actions to improve the services in order to reach objectives such as World Health Organization's sustainable development goals [22].

In any organization, each and every activity is aimed to transform and increase the value of an entry. Such processes may be effective if the objective is reached or efficient if the result is made using the least amount of resources. Both concepts are related to the performance of the organization.

In spite of the importance of the performance, it is not obvious to estimate. Since data envelopment analysis is a quantitative robust tool to determine the efficiency, its applications and importance are substantial. Seddhigi et al. cited a systematic review of 137 papers by Hafidz et al. who found that the most would employ data envelopment analysis for measuring efficiency in health systems [8,17].

© ICST Institute for Computer Sciences, Social Informatics and Telecommunications Engineering 2021
Published by Springer Nature Switzerland AG 2021. All Rights Reserved
J. A. Marmolejo-Saucedo et al. (Eds.): COMPSE 2021, LNICST 393, pp. 162–173, 2021.
https://doi.org/10.1007/978-3-030-87495-7_11

The measurement of efficiency is fundamental in health systems. Given its importance, there are many works related to this topic in the literature. Comparing international health systems, [16] proposes an analysis to evaluate health equity in terms of health outcomes, in international comparative analysis. At the continental level, various comparisons of health systems have been made. In [2,7,12] DEA models are used to compare the health systems of the member states of the European Union with different approaches. Similar analyses are proposed in Asia, Africa in [18,19] and the Visegrád Group [10].

However, it is more common to compare national system entities, e.g., a DEA assessment of health systems in the United States is presented in [6]. In China, [3,4,23–25] evaluate efficiency through DEA and other tools, such as regression analysis and game theory. In [5,11,14,15,20] the technique is used to compare the health systems of Portugal, the Czech Republic, Panama, Poland, and Brazil, respectively.

Considering the COVID-19 pandemic, there are some works that compare the efficiency of some international health systems considering variables that are measured worldwide: medical personnel (doctors and nurses), hospital beds, COVID-19 tests performed, cases affected, cases recovered, and cases of deaths [13].

This paper presents a comparison of the efficiency of international health systems, with a special focus on the countries of the American continent.

2   Data Envelopment Analysis

Data Envelopment Analysis compares the performance of different entities called decision-making units (DMUs) by using a set of n observations, m inputs, and s outputs of the process analyzed. These observations should be chosen wisely so they can describe the phenomena. It is recommended the number of DMU is at least 2 or 3 times the number of observations [26].

This method builds a frontier of best practices aimed to surround the non-efficient ones. This can be achieved by a straight line (constant return-to-scale, CRS) or by the linking of various points through line segments so a more approximated curve can be built (variable return-to-scale, VRS), which implies more accuracy (see Fig. 1) [9].

Since DEA is a linear programming application, even though the objective will be the same, the variables involved may be considered by two approaches, both of interest:

- Additive model (primal): determines the quantity of each observation.
- Multiplicative model (dual): determines the importance of each observation.

2.1   Additive VRS Model

DEA additive VRS model either minimizes the inputs or maximizes the outputs, only one approach can be taken while fixing the complement. Observe models (1) and (2), where both θ and ϕ are the efficiencies achieved in two different

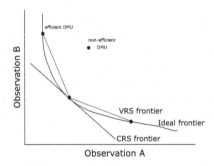

Fig. 1. Frontiers of efficiencies or good practices where de efficient DMUs are and that surround the non-efficient ones. Note the differences between the ideal, the CRS and the VRS frontier. (Own creation).

cases. Note in the model (1) θ is to be minimized since is input-oriented, the inputs are variables and the outputs cannot be modified, i.e. the decision is how to set the entries to achieve a specific output. Similarly, ϕ should be maximized since it is the output-oriented model and defines the best set of outputs obtained from fixed inputs. Deciding which model to use is essential to obtain meaningful results.

$$\theta^* = \min \theta \qquad\qquad \phi^* = \max \phi$$

subject to: subject to:

$$\sum_{j=1}^{n} \lambda_j x_{ij} \leq \theta x_{io} \qquad i = 1, 2, ..., m \qquad\qquad \sum_{j=1}^{n} \lambda_j x_{ij} \leq x_{io} \qquad i = 1, 2, ..., m$$

$$\sum_{j=1}^{n} \lambda_j y_{rj} \geq y_{ro} \qquad r = 1, 2, ..., s \quad (1) \qquad \sum_{j=1}^{n} \lambda_j y_{rj} \geq \phi y_{ro} \qquad r = 1, 2, ..., s \quad (2)$$

$$\sum_{j=1}^{n} \lambda_j = 1 \qquad j = 1, 2, ..., n \qquad\qquad \sum_{j=1}^{n} \lambda_j = 1 \qquad j = 1, 2, ..., n$$

$$\lambda_j \geq 0 \qquad\qquad\qquad\qquad\qquad \lambda_j \geq 0$$

Where θ, ϕ are the efficiencies of the input and output models respectively,

x_{ij} is the i-th input of the DMU_j,
y_{rj} is the r-th output of the DMU_j,
λ_j is the level of service achievable by the j-th DMU.

Please note that DMU_o refers to a specific DMU, so this model should be written n times so each and every DMU is compared with the rest ($o = 1, 2, ..., n$). In addition, note that the ideal value of both θ and ϕ is 1 (efficient). In other case, we could find $\theta < 1$ or $\phi > 1$.

The value of λ_j is relevant since it represents a benchmark of service for the DMU studied. For instance, for the DMU_o with $\lambda_a = \lambda_b = 0.5(a, b \neq o)$ would not be efficient since $\lambda_o \neq 1$ and its benchmarks to improve the fastest would be DMU_a and DMU_b.

2.2 Multiplicative VRS Model

The multiplicative models aim to identify the importance of each observation. Observe models (3) and (4), input and output-oriented, respectively. A set of weights are defined, u_r is the importance of the r-th input whereas v_i is to the i-th output. Note this model has n restrictions ($j = 1, 2, ..., n$) instead of the $m + s$ restrictions the primal model has. [9] The free variables u_0, v_0 are slacks, so a zero value of them might be related to an efficient DMU.

$$\max \sum_{r=1}^{s} u_r y_{ro} + u_0$$

$$\text{s. t.: } -\sum_{i=1}^{m} v_i x_{ij} + \sum_{r=1}^{s} u_r y_{rj} + u_0 \leq 0 \quad (3)$$

$$\sum_{i=1}^{m} v_i x_{io} = 1$$

$$u_r, v_i \geq 0$$

$$\min \sum_{i=1}^{m} v_i x_{io} + v_0$$

$$\text{s. t.: } \sum_{i=1}^{m} v_i x_{ij} - \sum_{r=1}^{s} u_r y_{rj} + v_0 \leq 0 \quad (4)$$

$$\sum_{i=1}^{m} u_i y_{ro} = 1$$

$$u_r, v_i \geq 0$$

This step gives important feedback about the observations considered so corrections can be made, such as deleting or adding observations [1].

2.3 Slacks

VRS models can identify efficient DMUs. However, they could be strongly or weakly efficient (see Fig. 2). Therefore, a second stage should be implemented which is to find the slacks, that are tolerances acceptable for each DMU, reducing inputs (s_i^-) or increasing outputs (s_r^+).

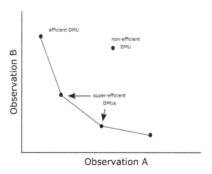

Fig. 2. Efficient and super-efficient DMUs located on the frontier. Note in this case an equilibrium of both observations A and B used are related to a super-efficient DMU. (Own creation).

Observe models (5) and (6), input and output-oriented, respectively. In both cases, the objective is to maximize the slacks. Note the efficiencies are fixed [26].

$$\max \quad \sum_{i=1}^{m} s_i^- + \sum_{r=1}^{s} s_r^+ \qquad\qquad \max \quad \sum_{i=1}^{m} s_i^- + \sum_{r=1}^{s} s_r^+$$

$$\text{s. t.:} \quad \sum_{j=1}^{n} \lambda_j x_{ij} + s_i^- = \theta^* x_{io} \qquad \text{s. t.:} \quad \sum_{j=1}^{n} \lambda_j x_{ij} + s_i^- = x_{io}$$

$$\sum_{j=1}^{n} \lambda_j y_{rj} - s_r^+ = y_{ro} \quad (5) \qquad \sum_{j=1}^{n} \lambda_j y_{rj} - s_r^+ = \phi^* y_{ro} \quad (6)$$

$$\sum_{j=1}^{n} \lambda_j = 1 \qquad\qquad \sum_{j=1}^{n} \lambda_j = 1$$

$$\lambda_j \geq 0 \qquad\qquad \lambda_j \geq 0$$

If certain DMU results to have $\theta, \phi = 1$ and $s_i^{-*} = s_r^{+*} = 0$ for all i and r, we can say it is super-efficient.

3   Application

The selected model is the output-oriented VRS in order to obtain the best results by using a fixed set of inputs. The data processing was done through an own written R script, based on Hosseinzadeh et al.'s code [9], which uses the package 'lpSolve' to solve for every DMU. The script results were also verified with the R package 'deaR'.

3.1   Data

The observations chosen for the 39 healthcare systems are shown in Table 1. The data selected was the most recently reported by each country between the years 2016 and 2019 [21], since the changes are not drastic and the model does not allow empty spaces (see Table 2).

Table 1. Observations chosen for evaluating the performance of a healthcare system.

Observation	Alias	Description
Inputs	Health kUSD	Health expenditure in 1000 USD per capita
	Beds	Hospital beds per thousand people
	Physicians	Physicians per thousand people
	Nurses	Nurses and midwives per thousand people
Outputs	Life Exp	Life expectancy at birth
	Disease Deaths	Diseases deaths per thousand (from communicable and non-communicable deaths)
	MCCDR	Mortality from cardiovascular diseases, cancer, diabetes or chronic respiratory diseases (percentage)
	Diabetes	Percentage of diabetes prevalence

Table 2. Data set built for healthcare systems evaluation. Note some of the outputs are negative since they should be minimized instead of maximized.

Country	Health kUSD	Beds	Physicians	Nurses	Life Exp	Disease Deaths	MCCDR	Diabetes
Argentina	1.12790723	4.99	3.9901	2.5996	76.667	−7.169884	−15.7	−5.9
Austria	5.32643701	7.27	5.1697	7.0899	81.7926829	−8.8881403	−10.4	−6.6
Belgium	4.91270068	5.62	3.0709	19.4614	81.7463415	−8.9185082	−10.6	−4.6
Bolivia	0.22359789	1.29	1.5901	1.5589	71.513	−6.1735856	−17.9	−6.8
Brazil	0.84838885	2.09	2.1643	10.119	75.881	−5.7764304	−15.5	−10.4
Canada	4.99490234	2.55	2.6102	9.9438	82.0487805	−7.1881473	−9.6	−7.6
Chile	1.45560791	2.06	2.5912	13.3248	80.181	−5.7684861	−10	−8.6
China	0.50105939	4.31	1.9798	2.6621	76.912	−6.6159779	−15.9	−9.2
Colombia	0.51315869	1.71	2.1848	1.3309	77.287	−4.8409828	−9.7	−7.4
Cuba	0.98693732	5.33	8.4218	7.5614	78.802	−8.4620948	−16.6	−9.6
Denmark	6.21676855	2.43	4.0099	10.3195	81.202439	−8.9730103	−10.8	−8.3
Ecuador	0.51624799	1.39	2.0368	2.5059	77.01	−4.5341484	−11	−5.5
Finland	4.51567725	3.61	3.8118	14.7374	81.7853659	−9.2469853	−9.6	−5.6
France	4.69007227	5.91	3.2672	11.4707	82.5780488	−8.521616	−10.6	−4.8
Germany	5.47220215	8	4.2488	13.2352	80.9414634	−10.77549	−12.1	−10.4
Greece	1.5668999	4.2	5.4789	3.6331	81.9390244	−11.242621	−12.5	−4.7
Hungary	1.08180286	7.01	3.4075	6.9157	76.0219512	−12.749754	−22.1	−6.9
Iceland	6.53093213	2.87	4.0778	16.2132	82.5609756	−5.9496626	−8.7	−5.8
Ireland	5.4890708	2.97	3.3125	16.0996	82.302439	−6.0536993	−9.7	−3.2
Italy	2.98899585	3.14	3.9774	5.7401	83.197561	−10.095046	−9	−5
Japan	4.26658691	12.98	2.4115	12.1531	84.3563415	−10.554673	−8.3	−5.6
Korea, Rep.	2.54281812	12.43	2.3608	7.3009	83.2268293	−5.1721349	−7.3	−6.9
Luxembourg	6.22708398	4.51	3.009	12.1744	82.4463415	−6.4827734	−9.7	−5
Mexico	0.51960547	0.98	2.3827	2.3961	75.054	−5.4436178	−15.6	−13.5
Netherlands	5.30653467	3.17	3.6054	11.1839	82.0121951	−8.2926811	−10.3	−5.4
Norway	8.2390957	3.53	2.9164	18.2248	82.9073171	−7.17453	−8.7	−5.3
Paraguay	0.40039273	0.83	1.3544	1.6604	74.254	−4.9237504	−16	−9.6
Poland	0.97873566	6.54	2.3788	6.8926	77.8560976	−10.341985	−17	−6.1
Portugal	2.21517358	3.45	5.124	6.9746	80.6829268	−10.377485	−11	−9.8
Singapore	2.82363818	2.49	2.2936	6.2432	83.497561	−4.7863234	−9.5	−5.5
Spain	2.73632324	2.97	3.8723	5.7295	83.4853659	−8.4812551	−9.6	−6.9
Sweden	5.98170605	2.14	3.984	11.8164	82.9585366	−8.1667783	−8.4	−4.8
United Arab Emirates	1.81734766	1.38	2.5278	5.7271	77.972	−1.2805499	−18.5	−16.3
United Kingdom	4.31542773	2.5	2.8117	8.1723	81.204878	−8.6682466	−10.3	−3.9
United States	10.6238496	2.87	2.612	14.548	78.7878049	−8.1298925	−13.6	−10.8
Uruguay	1.59004822	2.43	5.0794	1.9412	77.911	−8.7780898	−16.5	−7.3
Australia	5.42534033	3.84	3.6778	12.5508	82.9	−6.3017123	−8.6	−5.6
Russian Federation	0.60900916	7.12	4.0139	8.5429	73.0839024	−12.396768	−24.2	−6.1
Saudi Arabia	1.48459338	2.24	2.6117	5.4763	75.133	−2.8229543	−20.9	−15.8

3.2 Results

The next tables summarizes the results obtained. Table 3 shows super-efficient healthcare systems, which means that resulted in values $\phi = 1, \sum \text{Slacks} = 0$. Both Tables 3 and 6, for super-efficient and inefficient DMUs respectively, show the weights related to each observation, shoeing which aspects deserve to be enhanced and how remarkable the improvement would be.

Table 3. Weights of super-efficient healthcare systems. All these DMUs had $\phi = 1$ and $\sum Slacks = 0$.

DMU	v_1	v_2	v_3	v_4	u_1	u_2	u_3	u_4	v_0
Bolivia	0	0	0.62889126	0	0.02335976	0	0.00688633	0.08047957	0
Chile	0.02937194	0.01087341	0	0.00036444	0.01250012	0	0	0.00026421	0.92999067
China	0.03617291	0	0.02164895	0	0.01300187	0	0	0	0.93901463
Colombia	0	0.0057436	0	0.01544373	0.01912439	0	0.0492852	0	
Ecuador	0.00226697	0	0.49039164	0	0.02832821	0.20865524	0	0.04281484	0
Greece	0.04172753	0	0.02714084	0.00072401	0.01633238	0	0	0.07197	0.78328481
Iceland	0	0.15699239	0.13473732	0	0.10483232	0.17871106	0.75767679	0	0
Ireland	0	0.00074946	0	0.00034392	0.01246554	0	0	0.00810757	0.99223709
Italy	0	0.0159608	0.18009223	0.04069341	0.06434565	0	0.30723874	0.31765058	0
Japan	0	0	0.41467966	0	0.0166026	0	0.03099295	0.02558798	0
Korea, Rep.	0	0	0.42358523	0	0.01591407	0	0.02678758	0.01868521	0
Norway	0	0.03817635	0.26707947	0.00473678	0.05881405	0	0.32063066	0.20502419	0
Paraguay	0	0	0.20652898	0	0.01523049	0	0.00818278	0	0.72027715
Singapore	0.02692634	0	0.40284694	0	0.02351959	0.13809514	0.03188004	0	0
Spain	0.01710778	0.00015162	0.00080757	0	0.01197815	0	0	0	0.94961011
Sweden	0	0.01295001	0.14612027	0.03301715	0.05220772	0	0.2492823	0.2577301	0
United Arab Emirates	0	0	0.39560092	0	0.02078241	0.12336022	0.02499875	0	0
United Kingdom	0.01866848	0	0.32700414	0	0.01958365	0	0	0.15135586	0

Tables 4 and 5 show the efficiencies determined, the sum of the slacks found (which should be zero), the closest countries as a benchmark, and the factor of each benchmark.

Table 4. Efficiencies, slacks and benchmarks for Americas' inefficient healthcare systems.

DMU	Efficiency	SumSlacks	Benchmark	Factor
Argentina	1.03747931	8.15158435	Colombia	0.49867127
			Ecuador	0.03457781
			Greece	0.40793435
			Singapore	0.05881656
Brazil	1.02963524	18.9580786	Colombia	0.58704971
			Ecuador	0.26395383
			Korea, Rep.	0.03503501
			Singapore	0.11396145
Canada	1.01771742	11.1529506	Japan	0.00571973
			Singapore	0.99428027
Cuba	1.00731737	22.5032809	Colombia	0.55038427
			Greece	0.44961573
Mexico	1.00008846	6.65982428	Ecuador	0.20139955
			Paraguay	0.73093454
			United Arab Emirates	0.06766591
United States	1.06017258	30.6846495	Japan	0.03622498
			Singapore	0.96377502
Uruguay	1.0078195	12.0471215	Colombia	0.73490574
			Greece	0.26509426

Table 5. Efficiencies, slacks and referents for other non-efficient countries.

DMU	Efficiency	SumSlacks	Benchmark	Factor
Australia	1.00180085	2.9509122	Iceland	0.23388361
			Korea, Rep.	0.13938215
			Singapore	0.27149325
			Sweden	0.35524099
Austria	1.02294997	7.66540688	Japan	0.21178156
			Spain	0.78821844
Belgium	1.01903834	12.8123944	Ireland	0.36547358
			Japan	0.28165612
			Singapore	0.3528703
Denmark	1.02712625	16.176426	Singapore	0.82857143
			Sweden	0.17142857
Finland	1.02205634	15.6082404	Japan	0.10676835
			Singapore	0.89323165
France	1.0100877	4.87862012	Ireland	0.2968796
			Japan	0.31244021
			Singapore	0.3906802
Germany	1.03715256	19.9449911	Japan	0.52526215
			Singapore	0.47473785
Hungary	1.0460887	27.2097128	Colombia	0.54367037
			Greece	0.36637247
			Korea, Rep.	0.08995716
Luxembourg	1.0117648	6.93016513	Ireland	0.19979053
			Japan	0.18342236
			Singapore	0.61678711
Netherlands	1.01875637	12.5774589	Ireland	0.0022555
			Japan	0.06472043
			Singapore	0.93302406
Poland	1.00978297	18.7353922	Colombia	0.23593181
			Ecuador	0.501223
			Greece	0.07117163
			Korea, Rep.	0.19167357
Portugal	1.02596818	9.23842065	Greece	0.45875483
			Singapore	0.17555925
			Spain	0.36568592
Russian Federation	1.0618778	36.6087166	Colombia	0.55230794
			Ecuador	0.35777893
			Greece	0.08991314
Saudi Arabia	1.04366239	13.3423767	Colombia	0.33825606
			Korea, Rep.	0.06134861
			Singapore	0.06348956
			United Arab Emirates	0.53690578

Table 6. Observation weights for inefficient healthcare systems.

DMU	Weights							
	Inputs				Outputs			
	Health kUSD	Beds	Physicians	Nurses	Life Exp	Disease Deaths	MCCDR	Diabetes
Argentina	0	0	0	0.02570587	0.01515057	0.0088022	0	0.01668436
Australia	0	0.00789764	0	0	0.01702046	0.01102571	0.03971106	0
Austria	0	0	0	0.00165773	0.01222603	0	0	0
Belgium	0	0.00096819	0	0	0.01261314	0	0	0.00675607
Brazil	0.03412508	0.00044001	0.02442616	0	0.01317853	0	0	0
Canada	0	0.00099778	0	0	0.01218787	0	0	0
Cuba	0.05602357	0	0	0	0.01269003	0	0	0
Denmark	0	0.01896581	0	0	0.0123149	0	0	0
Finland	0	0.00100099	0	0	0.01222713	0	0	0
France	0	0.00095942	0	0	0.01249891	0	0	0.00669489
Germany	0	0.00101143	0	0	0.01235461	0	0	0
Hungary	0.03793714	0	0.00644098	0	0.0131541	0	0	0
Luxembourg	0	0.00096229	0	0	0.01253633	0	0	0.00671493
Mexico	0.01033877	0.06343291	0	0	0.01332374	0	0	0
Netherlands	0	0.00097018	0	0	0.01263907	0	0	0.00676996
Poland	0.03760151	0	0.00738879	0	0.01295185	0	0	0.00137383
Portugal	0.019857	0.00329722	0	0	0.0123942	0	0	0
United States	0	0.00103908	0	0	0.01269232	0	0	0
Uruguay	0	0	0	0.02593583	0.01283516	0	0	0
Russian Federation	0.06664677	0	0	0	0.01386061	0	0	0.0021291
Saudi Arabia	0.03705213	0.00024966	0	0	0.01371963	0.01090953	0	0

4   Conclusion

Observing both the value of the efficiency and the sum of the slacks, it is noticeable that the context of Mexico is not so privileged, since the system is already collapsed due to the economical situation of this country.

It might be feasible to increase Mexico's attention to the healthcare systems of Ecuador, Paraguay, and United Arab Emirates, as Table 4 shows. Particularly, the health expenditure and beds per thousand people could be enhanced so an improvement in the life expectancy at birth is noticeable. Similar inferences for any of the countries studied can be made from these results.

5   Discussion

This analysis may be more robust if more indicators are considered and could show more representative information as the data is more recent. In future analysis, not only could more countries be added but it could also be possible to take into account more observations related to the World Health Organization's sustainable development goals [22] such as the equality of the services given all economic strata or the total of population health-covered.

Acknowledgements. This research has been funded by National Autonomous University of Mexico as the project PAPIIT IA105220 Optimización en la logística hospitalaria.

References

1. Bonilla, M., Casasús, T., Medal, A., Sala, R.: Un Análisis de la Eficiencia de los Puertos Españoles. VI Jornada de ASEPUMA, Ud Valencia, Departamento de Economía Financiera y Matemática: Santiago de Compostela (97), 9 (1998)
2. Briestensky, R., Kljucnikov, A.: "The impact of DRG-based management of healthcare facilities on amenable mortality in the European union. Prob. Perspect. Manag. **19**(2), 264–275 (2021). https://doi.org/10.21511/ppm.19(2). 2021.22. https://www.scopus.com/inward/record.uri?eid=2-s2.0-85109032676&doi=10.21511%2fppm.19%282%29.2021.22&partnerID=40&md5=102d0d2b3371321 e4074cb303e6f5a25. Cited By 0
3. Chai, P., Wan, Q., Kinfu, Y.: Efficiency and productivity of health systems in prevention and control of non-communicable diseases in China, 2008–2015. Eur. J. Health Econ. **22**(2), 267–279 (2021). https://doi.org/10.1007/s10198-020-01251-3. https://www.scopus.com/inward/record.uri?eid=2-s2.0-85098692749&doi=10.1007%2fs10198-020-01251-3&partnerID=40&md5=3bc310b679b925cba13246 c31bdf019a. Cited By 0
4. Chen, Z., Chen, X., Gan, X., Bai, K., Baležentis, T., Cui, L.: Technical efficiency of regional public hospitals in China based on the three-stage DEA. Int. J. Environ. Res. Public Health **17**(24), 1–17 (2020). https://doi.org/10.3390/ijerph17249383. https://www.scopus.com/inward/record.uri?eid=2-s2.0-85097940247&doi=10.339 0%2fijerph17249383&partnerID=40&md5=e913fd7d29d2994fbde6653560a66498. Cited By 0
5. Cordero, J., García-García, A., Lau-Cortés, E., Polo, C.: Assessing panamanian hospitals' performance with alternative frontier methods. Int. Trans. Oper. Res. (2021). https://doi.org/10.1111/itor.13013. https://www.scopus.com/inward/ record.uri?eid=2-s2.0-85107204634&doi=10.1111%2fitor.13013&partnerID=40& md5=a5614354ec137d87b8a5ef893dc6132c. Cited By 0
6. Darabi, N., Ebrahimvandi, A., Hosseinichimeh, N., Triantis, K.: A DEA evaluation of U.S. STATES' healthcare systems in terms of their birth outcomes. Expert Syst. Appl. **182** (2021). https://doi.org/10.1016/j.eswa.2021.115278. https:// www.scopus.com/inward/record.uri?eid=2-s2.0-85107660523&doi=10.1016%2fj. eswa.2021.115278&partnerID=40&md5=b8f3cb48a329b94c6469d01c92a99b1c. Cited By 0
7. Dincă, G., Dincăp, M., Andronic, M.: The efficiency of the healthcare systems in EU countries - a DEA analysis. Acta Oeconomica **70**(1), 19–36 (2020). https://doi.org/10.1556/032.2020.00002. https://www.scopus.com/inward/record. uri?eid=2-s2.0-85089176349&doi=10.1556%2f032.2020.00002&partnerID=40& md5=ada2b82b7953ecdfa36ec6650957e1d8. Cited By 3
8. Hafidz, F., Ensor, T., Tubeuf, S.: Efficiency measurement in health facilities: a systematic review in low- and middle-income countries. Appl. Health Econ. Health Policy **16**(4), 465–480 (2018). https://doi.org/10.1007/s40258-018-0385-7
9. Hosseinzadeh Lotfi, F., Ebrahimnejad, A., Vaez-Ghasemi, M., Moghaddas, Z.: Data Envelopment Analysis with R. In: Studies in Fuzziness and Soft Computing, vol. 386. Springer, Cham (2020). https://doi.org/10.1007/978-3-030-24277-0. http://link.springer.com/10.1007/978-3-030-24277-0
10. Lacko, R., Markovič, P., Šagátová, S., Hajduová, Z.: Evaluation and development of environmental and health efficiency: Case of v4 countries. Ekonomicky casopis **68**(10), 1040–1056 (2020). https://doi.org/10.31577/ekoncas.2020.10.04. https://www.scopus.com/inward/record.uri?eid=2-s2.0-85099049479&doi=10.315

77%2fekoncas.2020.10.04&partnerID=40&md5=2e62fa928153929d82157ac27221c e48. Cited By 0

11. Miszczynska, K., Miszczyński, P.: Measuring the efficiency of the healthcare sector in Poland – a window-DEA evaluation. Int. J. Prod. Perform. Manag. (2021). https://doi.org/10.1108/IJPPM-06-2020-0276. https://www.scopus.com/inward/record.uri?eid=2-s2.0-85103404006&doi=10.1108%2fIJPPM-06-2020-0276&partnerID=40&md5=6ba82e76e0113a91dd764dbe8d130907. Cited By 0

12. Mitropoulos, P.: Production and quality performance of healthcare services in EU countries during the economic crisis. Oper. Res. **21**(2), 857–873 (2021). https://doi.org/10.1007/s12351-019-00483-3. https://www.scopus.com/inward/record.uri?eid=2-s2.0-85081212915&doi=10.1007%2fs12351-019-00483-3&partnerID=40&md5=4a591d9780af0bc0b8211b1247e01d0e. Cited By 3

13. Mourad, N., Habib, A., Tharwat, A.: Appraising healthcare systems' efficiency in facing COVID-19 through data envelopment analysis. Decis. Sci. Lett. **10**(3), 301–310 (2021). https://doi.org/10.5267/j.dsl.2021.2.007. https://www.scopus.com/inward/record.uri?eid=2-s2.0-85106921537&doi=10.5267%2fj.dsl.2021.2.007&partnerID=40&md5=0503bfbcf5438b789c143511b114df22. Cited By 0

14. Peixoto, M., Musetti, M., Mendonça, M.: Performance management in hospital organizations from the perspective of principal component analysis and data envelopment analysis: the case of federal university hospitals in Brazil. Comput. Ind. Eng. **150** (2020). https://doi.org/10.1016/j.cie.2020.106873. https://www.scopus.com/inward/record.uri?eid=2-s2.0-85092105354&doi=10.1016%2fj.cie.2020.106873&partnerID=40&md5=317a648c569e18bdbedf72cf7c022e05. Cited By 2

15. Pereira, M., Ferreira, D., Figueira, J., Marques, R.: Measuring the efficiency of the Portuguese public hospitals: a value modelled network data envelopment analysis with simulation. Expert Syst. Appl. **181** (2021). https://doi.org/10.1016/j.eswa.2021.115169. https://www.scopus.com/inward/record.uri?eid=2-s2.0-85105546492&doi=10.1016%2fj.eswa.2021.115169&partnerID=40&md5=a56fedf4cb9be0b8a8ea06b2c773481c. Cited By 0

16. Schenkman, S., Bousquat, A.: From income inequality to social inequity: impact on health levels in an international efficiency comparison panel. BMC Public Health **21**(1) (2021). https://doi.org/10.1186/s12889-021-10395-7. https://www.scopus.com/inward/record.uri?eid=2-s2.0-85104017932&doi=10.1186%2fs12889-021-10395-7&partnerID=40&md5=41f5bd5fb581517805522e4a4171f068. Cited By 0

17. Seddighi, H., Nosrati Nejad, F., Basakha, M.: Health systems efficiency in Eastern Mediterranean region: a data envelopment analysis. Cost Effectiveness Resour. Allocat. **18**(1), 1–8 (2020). https://doi.org/10.1186/s12962-020-00217-9

18. Singh, S., Bala, M., Kumar, N., Janor, H.: Application of DEA-based malmquist productivity index on health care system efficiency of Asian countries. Int. J. Health Plan. Manag. (2021). https://doi.org/10.1002/hpm.3169. https://www.scopus.com/inward/record.uri?eid=2-s2.0-85104241429&doi=10.1002%2fhpm.3169&partnerID=40&md5=6c2738b303ea271233d40cff35a90140. Cited By 0

19. Top, M., Konca, M., Sapaz, B.: Technical efficiency of healthcare systems in African countries: an application based on data envelopment analysis. Health Policy Technol. **9**(1), 62–68 (2020). https://doi.org/10.1016/j.hlpt.2019.11.010. https://www.scopus.com/inward/record.uri?eid=2-s2.0-85076592553&doi=10.1016%2fj.hlpt.2019.11.010&partnerID=40&md5=9290dd4249f562548f2b89698589ab6d. Cited By 8

20. Vrabková, I., Vaňková, I.: Efficiency of human resources in public hospitals: an example from the Czech Republic. Int. J. Environ. Res. Public Health **18**(9) (2021). https://doi.org/10.3390/ijerph18094711. https://www.scopus.com/inward/record.uri?eid=2-s2.0-85104794289&doi=10.3390%2fijerph18094711&partnerID=40&md5=d196ba0c724695b904b1547d4f90eb64. Cited By 0

21. World Data Bank: Health Nutrition and Population Statistics—DataBank. https://databank.worldbank.org/source/health-nutrition-and-population-statistics

22. World Health Organization: World Health Statistics - Monitoring Health For The SDGs. World Health Organization, p. 1.121 (2016)

23. Yaya, S., Xi, C., Xiaoyang, Z., Meixia, Z.: Evaluating the efficiency of China's healthcare service: a weighted DEA-game theory in a competitive environment. J. Clean. Prod. **270** (2020). https://doi.org/10.1016/j.jclepro.2020.122431. https://www.scopus.com/inward/record.uri?eid=2-s2.0-85087743297&doi=10.1016%2fj.jclepro.2020.122431&partnerID=40&md5=5dce288ebf0b59042c3552195b76a585. Cited By 3

24. Yu, J., Liu, Z., Zhang, T., Hatab, A., Lan, J.: Measuring productivity of healthcare services under environmental constraints: evidence from China. BMC Health Serv. Res. **20**(1) (2020). https://doi.org/10.1186/s12913-020-05496-9. https://www.scopus.com/inward/record.uri?eid=2-s2.0-85088425147&doi=10.1186%2fs12913-020-05496-9&partnerID=40&md5=91a7ccfe76ba0ca38d7016c6fb033455. Cited By 2

25. Zhang, T., Lu, W., Tao, H.: Efficiency of health resource utilisation in primary-level maternal and child health hospitals in Shanxi province, China: a bootstrapping data envelopment analysis and truncated regression approach. BMC Health Serv. Res. **20**(1) (2020). https://doi.org/10.1186/s12913-020-5032-y. https://www.scopus.com/inward/record.uri?eid=2-s2.0-85081199838&doi=10.1186%2fs12913-020-5032-y&partnerID=40&md5=4327aa0194a9e3ad5ec827138cb4db18. Cited By 6

26. Zhu, J.: Quantitative Models for Performance Evaluation and Benchmarking. In: International Series in Operations Research & Management Science, vol. 213. Springer, Cham (2014). https://doi.org/10.1007/978-3-319-06647-9. http://link.springer.com/10.1007/978-3-319-06647-9

Industry 4.0 in Logistics and Supply Chain

Organizational Efficiency in the Implementation of 4.0 Technologies in Logistics Operators in the Colombian Caribbean Region

Jania Astrid Saucedo-Martinez[1], Carlos Jose Regalao-Noriega[2(✉)], and Luis Ortiz-Ospino[2]

[1] Facultad de Ingenieria Mecanica y Electrica, Universidad Autonoma de Nuevo Leon, Ciudad Universitaria, San Nicolas de los Garza, Nuevo Leon, Mexico
jania.saucedomrt@uanl.edu.mx
[2] Facultad de Ingenierias, Universidad SimonBolivar, Barranquilla, Atlantico, Colombia
{cregalao,lortiz27}@unisimonbolivar.edu.co

Abstract. Logistics operators in Colombian Caribbean region structure their activities based on the grouping of processes linked to intralogistics activities. Consequently, this project aims to demonstrate that the improvement in the organizational efficiency index of these organizations should be developed through the implementation of 4.0 technologies, using the strengths provided by the implementation of simulation concepts in decision-making tool for intralogistics activities in logistics operators on Colombian Caribbean region. For fulfillment of the objectives, literary research framed in three categories: intralogistics, technology 4.0 and business efficiency, and instruments to assess the efficiency indexes obtained with the application of the technologies 4.0 in the parent company object of study, to evaluate the supply chain based on intralogistics activities 4.0, using as method the research line of operations management as for the analysis of the thematic axis the supply chains based on intralogistics operations. To this end, a series of logical steps are established, starting from the perception and direct treatment to establish the elements involved in the measurement of efficiency in organizations based on decision-making according to the scenarios that allow determining the impact of technologies 4.0 and ending with evaluations of the same based on the theoretical average index, of the challenges and perspectives that the dynamics of the international system and especially the agreements of the international free trade treaties that the neo-grenadine nation has approved and materialized in the last decade to make its economy more fruitful and fundamentally to the organizations of its different regions.

Keywords: Intralogistics · Technologies 4.0 · Business efficiency

1 Introduction

Since the beginning of history, the human species has had to use its ingenuity to supply its basic needs, among the most important of which is food. To do so, they supplied

© ICST Institute for Computer Sciences, Social Informatics and Telecommunications Engineering 2021
Published by Springer Nature Switzerland AG 2021. All Rights Reserved
J. A. Marmolejo-Saucedo et al. (Eds.): COMPSE 2021, LNICST 393, pp. 177–195, 2021.
https://doi.org/10.1007/978-3-030-87495-7_12

this need with what was closest to the environment where they settled because at that time they did not yet have the knowledge of storage, distribution and transportation as methods of solution for their basic needs, the transport of provisions or goods was reduced to the amount that an individual or persons could mobilize and, consequently, the deposit of perishable provisions was only within reach for a short period, which forced citizens to settle near the sources of supply to take advantage of the goods and food that the environment could provide or that nature granted.

Even in the 21st century, in many parts of the planet, the consumption and production of goods at present only within specific geographical locations. Even today, there are worrying patterns in developing countries such as Asia, Latin America, Africa, and Australia, in which a group of its inhabitants lives reduced and autonomous spaces villages, where the consumer goods needed by the population are developed or managed in the vicinity of the settlements. By the above, it is evident that the logistical procedures are vital for the periodic activities of the individual or of a community in general, thus it follows that today's organizations explore multiple options in the field of management and administration of the supply chain of a set of diverse factors, rules and laws, from the most conservative dimensions of marketing, manufacturing, accounting, procurement and transportation, to the branches of applied mathematics, knowledge of organizational context and economic management, to respond to the demands of consumers on a global scale, following contemporary paradigms.

For this reason, the logistics work carried out within the communities has high relevance for the economic and social strengthening, especially of logistics operators and their supply chain. In some cases in the Caribbean region of Colombia, especially in the Atlantic, the subject of this study, the organization responsible for the permanent management of the various economic movements and industrialization, generating sources of employment and well-being for the residents, guaranteeing access to the items and accessories required to meet your expectations, with the influx of the Magdalena River as a primary factor, the needs described above are evident. Thus, the definition of the supply chainis as: "The supply chain, or simply supply chain, is a chain of suppliers, factories, warehouses, distribution centers, and retailers through which inputs are procured and transformed into products for delivery to the end customer" [1]. Intralogistics procedures of logistics operators represent almost thirty percent of the logistics costs of organizations in Colombia, which, according to the National Planning Department of Colombia, are equivalent to about fifteen percent of an organization's sales [2]. In the case of Colombia, there is no interference in the logistics sector, especially intralogistics, and these discrete steps in the organization are of great organizational importance and increase the cost of all products in the domestic market [3]. Following Crespo [4] "The costs derived from the logistics process, depending on the levels of the country, are at several percentage points of difference for the nations of America and Europe. For example, when compared to the United States, this represents 8.7% of the sales achieved, while in Europe it increases to 11.9% and in Latin America the estimate is around 14.7%".

Within the components, costs in Intralogistics are a predominant factor in the economies of all countries worldwide. For Colombia, we do not have data on how much this value represents for the whole logistics distribution and supply chain, but for

Brazil, for example, it represents an average of twenty-eight percent of the costs, that is, an important part of the value of an article to the final buyer, is concentrated in the processes derived between the creation of the final product and the final delivery to the client [5]. Consequently, to find instruments that tend to improve decision making that influence the indicators and, in turn, the factors that make up the organizational efficiency index in logistics operators, the aim is to find solutions to the challenge of inserting 4.0 technologies in intralogistics tasks, to achieve the purpose and respond to the problems of the organizations under study.

1.1 Requirements of Logistics Operators in the Colombian Caribbean Region

Under the problem statement, the purpose of this research focuses on: Improving the organizational efficiency index through the implementation of 4.0 technologies using simulation as a tool for decision making in intralogistics processes in the Colombian Caribbean region. The relationship items of the present research are aimed at establishing the following specific paragraphs:

i)   As a logistic operator in the Atlántico suite, carry out diagnostics of logistic and technical processes.
ii) Create simulation scenarios that facilitate the decision-making process for the implementation of technology in the internal operations of logistics operators in the Colombian Caribbean Atlantic.
iii) A statistical demonstration of the relevance of the research interests of this project as a reference in the implementation of technology in logistics processes.
iv) To evaluate the impact on the performance index of the organization of the internal processes of the logistics operators within the department of Atlántico through the investigated scenarios.

The current study is based on the consideration that the scenario assessment will provide greater certainty in decision-making regarding the application of technologies 4.0 in an overall context of comparing needs of the organization and will serve as an opening to a general development approach, the implementation, and evaluation of other areas of the industry in their intralogistics procedures. Organizational efficiency indices can be measured in those factors that influence decision-making, through the application of simulation in the intralogistics tasks or activities of logistics operators in the Colombian Caribbean region. The panorama of expansion of the logistic sector generates to us the requirement to incorporate new technologies, to understand and respond to the challenges of achieving sustainability in the market through the application of indices of continuous improvement in organizational efficiency, including the dynamics of the strategy and international standardization, as a fundamental aspect describing intelligent decision-making [6].

1.2 The Supply Chain in the Logistics Sector

Different authors establish the beginning of the study of logistics to military development Philippe-Pierre [7], Jordi [8], Roux [9], Ballou [10], Carranza [11]. This is primarily because the concept of logistics took its contemporary definition with the first theoretical evidence on military logistics at the end of World War I and achieved its greatest boom with the definition of logistics operation from a more complex and planned view of the time of the invasion of Europe in the development of World War II [10]. Accordingly, the relationship of logistic processes with military activities has been known since the beginning of the term logistics; during the end of the 4th century, treaties are evidenced by logistics in this military development. The agreements are justified by the logistics in this military advance. However, history shows other important non-military examples in the application of logistical skills such as the architecture of the pyramids in Egypt [12], who demystify their unique origin in the military branch and teach logistics as a discipline that took its first steps alongside the beginning of humanity and its social development [13].

Also, in the area of business, the description of the concept was established in 1844 by the French engineer Jules Dupuit who incorporated the notion of exchanging (Trade-off) a price for others and the selection among the different types of transport according to cost criteria [10]. The first writings that refer to logistics are evidenced in the year 1961 [14]. They capture the benefits of the planned logistics administration. Likewise, Drucker [15], highlighted the definition of logistics as one of the most important and last frontiers that enable real indicators of business efficiency and detailed it as "the dark continent of the economy" [12]. All these events gave rise to a growth in interest and development of the concept of logistics within the academic and business community. As a result, in 1962 the first association of logistics professionals, teachers, and managers was to promote education in this discipline and that there would be a reciprocity of ideas. The National Council of Physical Distribution Management (NCPDM), founded in 1963, officially defined logistics as "A set of activities that are responsible for the efficient movement of finished products from the end of the production line to the consumer and that, in some cases, includes the movement of raw materials from the source to the line" [16].

1.3 The Imperative Need to Improve Corporate Performance Indicators

The organizations that are organizing given the coming decade of the 21st century, are characterized by being companies that seek to achieve and demonstrate a better practice in their operations, mitigating the negative impact generated today by the lack of control of intralogistics activities within the supply chain and the absorption of the environment of technologies 4.0. The supply chain encompasses all aspects of business, people, the company, technology, and physical infrastructure that allows the innovation of inputs towards transformation into goods and services through management in different processes until deriving in the final product of value for a potential customer or consumer. He notes that this is a very functional vision, both internal and external to the company, which does not develop relationships of integration and synchronization, is perceived as an inventory of the elements of a system called the supply chain.

The comprehensive study on collaboration within the supply chain focuses on the development of various planning procedures and delimits multiple analyses in the information. Increasing the range of management schemes on different hierarchical levels, decision-making and empirical environments allow solutions to problems arising from intralogistics activities. The organizations that work in the Colombian Caribbean region, suffer these inconveniences in their intralogistics operations, Primarily logistics operators that show a considerable impact on their organizational efficiency index that in turn impacts on their productivity and competitiveness compared to different locations in the country and Latin America; the Colombian government under the leadership of President Iván Duque has framed the National Development Plan 2018–2022 called: "The Future Belongs to Everyone" and the strategic planning work of the Atlantic department of Governor Elsa Noguera: "Atlantic is the town", where it is added to the district strategic plans of the mayors of the cities of the department, include of primary relevance and rigorous compliance for the issue of logistics issues and their aspects as a fundamental aspect in the of productivity and competitiveness of the region and its companies.

Publications made worldwide, according to Botthof [19], establish that the costs of the logistic activities in the nations of Latin America and the Caribbean would contemplate a range between 50% and 80% more supported regarding the countries that are members of the Organization for Economic Cooperation and Development (OECD). Essentially in Colombia, due to the deviation of responsibility in the solution of the problems about road infrastructure, it admits the presence of a less efficient transport environment, poor quality in the management of the port environment through the appropriate use of capacity, and the minimum adaptation of other internal transport models, such as rail (used only for coal transport) or river transport, which also affects logistics operators. In this way, the BDI [20], argues that the logistics operators sector has a great opportunity for small and medium-sized enterprises, considering that logistics administration is part of the organization's most strategic activities, where the flow of costs that are formed is 19% of the Gross Domestic Product (GDP) in the countries of Latin America, evidenced especially by the complexity of customs processes among other elements. The inclusion of Information and Communication Technologies (ICT) in the area of Logistics in Colombia, remains in debt to increase the use of these technological advances, and specially to ensure that implementation determines a high impact of efficiency and effectiveness levels on logistics activities. Table 1 shows the demonstrated level of current inclusion of technologies in the logistics area and, specifically, their applicability in the logistics operators of the Colombian Caribbean region.

Information in the table above shows, using percentages, the degree of usability of technologies in intralogistics activities in the organizations above Colombian Caribbean region in accordance with the dynamics of the logistic field to total standards; the optimal level should be around 80% adaptability; however, we note that none of the technologies studied has reached international standards. For the foregoing, that the organizations in Colombia advance in modernization on the provision of logistics services, properly in the intralogistics activities of the sector, where relevant aspects are found such as infrastructure, performance indicators, management practices, and the increasing use of information systems to achieve organizational efficiency indices under the international standard.

Table 1. Applicable and applied technologies in Atlantic department logistics operators

ICTs in logistics operators	Available	Not Available
Optimization, planning and control of transport	57%	43%
Distribution Center Management (WMS)	28%	72%
Distribution Management System (DMS)	28%	72%
Business Transaction Management/Orders	28%	72%
Integrated WMS TMS	15%	85%
Demand management and planning software	24%	76%
ERP Interfaces	33%	67%
Fleet Management Software	45%	55%
Barcode system	24%	76%
Radiofrequency System	15%	85%
System for Invoicing/Auditor's	49%	51%
Real-time tracking and tracing system	73%	27%
Internet access for the client	63%	37%
Electronic Data Interchange System (EDI)	24%	76%
Picking Optimization System	15%	85%

2 Methodology

This research is framed in Operations Management in reference analysis of the thematic structure on the supply chain, about the intralogistics operations of logistics operators in the daily dynamics of the department of Atlántico in the Colombian Caribbean region. Through observation as a direct analysis activity evidence actions that impact decision-making in 4.0 technology implementation scenarios. Considering the above premise, a three-phase investigation is established:

i)   Starts with a full analysis of the current situation in the studied companies taking as a reference the analysis of vertical and horizontal integration systems in the framework of technology 4.0. Makes it possible to establish the current reality of the logistics operators in terms of the aspects under study in terms of their efficiency indexes.

ii) Then with the use of computational software and the application of Statistics, the possible scenarios for the analysis of the factors that will evaluate the impact of the parameters of the organizational efficiency index as the object of study of this research are specified.

iii) The results and evaluations according to the scenarios are quantitatively established according to the impact generated by implementing 4.0 technologies in the intralogistics processes on the improvement in organizational efficiency, using the procedure defined by Perez [23], which highlights three considerations in the characterization process: vertical and horizontal integration and, lastly, the use of technologies 4.0, as described in Table 2.

Table 2. Mapping the organizational structure

Consideration	Description
Vertical integration	It is based on the socio-technical system and the value creation modules
Horizontal integration	It is based on operations management requirements
Technologies 4.0	It contains the tools studied in the literature analysis
Scenario 1	Presents the current status of the organization under study
Scenario 2	Introduces organization with layout improvements
Scenario 3	Shows the implementation of technologies 4.0
Statistical field	Contains the tools for the analysis of the solution of the problem posed

The structure expressed in Table 2 is constituted as the starting point to know the current situation that the organization has in the study, i.e., evidence of the mechanisms and unfinished activities, loss events, and critical items of the operation, thus, the structured form of the instruments developed and applied in this research to analyses the current situation of logistics operators in the Colombian Caribbean region regarding the applicability of technologies 4.0; from the study of the aspects of vertical and horizontal integration, the creation of the three scenarios of analysis in the employability of the factors that determine the indicators of organizational efficiency, necessary steps for the solution of the problem studied.

This adaptation, developed by Perez [23] and Orozco [28], must be carried out strategically so that it responds satisfactorily to the requirements involved in intralogistics activities in the function of organizational efficiency. Taking into account the presented above, we can observe in Fig. 1 the results of the application of the tool of vertical and horizontal integration in the framework of applicability technologies 4.0 in the organization object of the present investigation, the parent company object of this research, which shows a ratio of vertical integration defined in 65%, delimited by the internal perception in the inclusion of 4.0 technologies and 64% of internal adaptation.

Figure 1 shows not only the diagnostic outcome of the integration and absorption of 4.0 technologies in the study organization but also details the individual characteristics of the organization and how they are adapting the inclusion of technologies, in the case of horizontal validation, it is evident that there is an opportunity gap for the adoption of emerging technologies, for such a case, it is shown that the external perception is around 59% of adaptability and the internal vision is 53%; on the other hand, the vertical validation shows us a different scenario of greater adaptation towards technological

Vertical and horizontal integration systems in the framework of industry 4.0: Evaluation and development

General Information

Type of evaluation		Responsible
Diagnosis	x	
Follow up		*Carlos Regalao Noriega*

Evaluators		Name of the organization:	*Logycem - Logistica al Dia*
Position held:	Quantity	Size of the organization People- Income	Type of organization:
Customer	4	Micro	Manufacturing x
Provider	4	Small	Technologies
Operational	2	Medium	Services
Director	1	Large x	

Diagnostic results

System evaluation

Vertical integration	65%	64%	Dif
Human	63%	62%	-1%
Human Integration	59%	51%	-8%
Administrative staff	63%	64%	1%
Operational personnel	66%	70%	4%
Organization	67%	68%	
Development and interrelations	70%	72%	2%
Information Management	63%	63%	0%
Team			
Cyber-physical interaction	59%	58%	-1%
Processes	64%	64%	
Development of operations	57%	55%	-2%
Lean Manufacturing	67%	70%	3%
Implementation of Core Tools	69%	67%	-1%
Product	67%	64%	
Research and Development	62%	59%	-2%
Technology	60%	58%	-2%
Sustainability	79%	75%	-4%

Horizontal integration	Dif.	59%	53%
Supply		64%	60%
Relationship Management	-5%	66%	61%
Information flow	-2%	60%	58%
Vendor evaluation	-7%	67%	61%
Comprehensive decisions	-2%	61%	59%
Planning and administration		52%	47%
Administration	-6%	63%	57%
Programming	-7%	41%	34%
Simulation	-2%	53%	50%
Customer Service		60%	58%
Order Management	-1%	45%	44%
Inventory Management	0%	63%	64%
Warehouse Management	-5%	70%	64%
Materials management	-5%	64%	59%
Transportation Management	-4%	59%	54%
Customer Service	-1%	61%	60%

Tools 4.0	61%	59%
Big data and analysis	61%	59%
Autonomous robots	62%	61%
Simulation	54%	52%
Integration systems	62%	60%
Industrial Internet of Things	61%	59%
Cybersecurity	60%	58%
3D manufacturing	63%	64%
Augmented reality	53%	48%
The Cloud	61%	59%
Advanced materials	79%	75%
Virtual Reality	62%	61%

Smooth perception (internal,
External perception
Difference

* External perception is excluded from internal processes

Fig. 1. Results of the application of the vertical and horizontal integration tool in the framework of applicability technologies 4.0

inclusion since it exceeds 60%, which leads to having a very good level of adaptation with favorable opportunities for improvement.

2.1 Scenario Analysis and Statistical Approximation

There are various ways to analyze the possible decisions that will lead us to a prosperous future, to put ourselves before the problems that can arise in an organization, and to identify aspects of continuous improvement, is what companies are looking for today; the above defines what this study puts into practice based on its methodological objective that consists in analyzing three scenarios through the applicability of the simulation as a means of analysis to define the impact generate the inclusion or absorption of technologies 4.0 organizations in the Colombian Caribbean region, specifically in logistics operators, to validate the increase or improvement of the organizational efficiency index, thus evidencing proposals in the implementation and analysis of solutions options to the problems of this research, shown in Fig. 2.

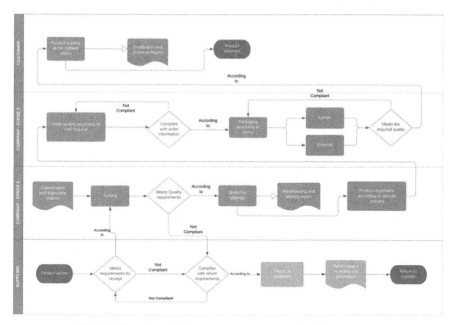

Fig. 2. Flowchart of the current process in the logistic operator

The main characteristic of intralogistics activity is the environment of storage, loading and unloading of raw materials as finished products or in transit depending on the nature and operation of the logistics operator. The above is specified in Fig. 2, where the operation of the warehouse to the other areas is evidenced, as well as the distribution process, loading, and unloading where the flow of products is centered, materials and skilled labor toward picking activities primarily, just as it is evident that the data generated is collected throughout the process, but there is no particular function for them other than to archive or save them.

Figure 3 shows the characteristics of the logistics operator with the operation factors framed in a different layout methodology, where it allows improving aspects of product reception and storage capacity, however, it does not allow giving an adequate solution to the finished product storage processes, since it maintains the results of the variables of the current scenario of the organization and the improvements in the loading and unloading process are not significant, impacting very little or nothing in the organizational efficiency index as shown in the analysis Table 4.

Figure 4 describes the functioning of the intralogistics processes of the logistics operator involving technology 4.0, in which substantial changes in the processes are evident. It details the results obtained by the logistics operator when applying this type of technology, the results according to the factors studied, and the gradual increase in organizational efficiency indicators, establishing the scenario as the ideal one for providing solutions to the problems of the logistics operators studied in this research project, represented in the analysis Table 3.

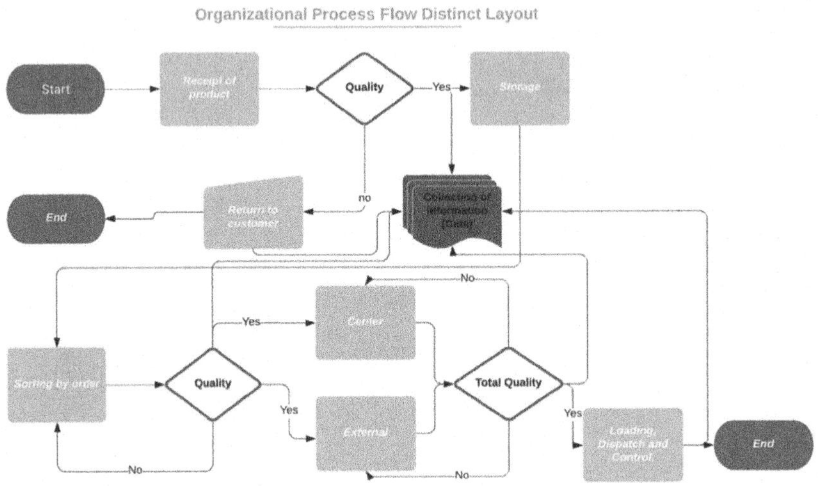

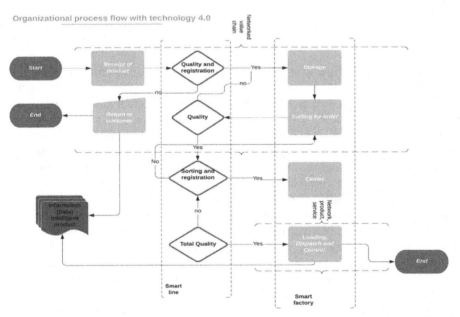

Fig. 3. Diagram of the intralogistics process within the organization's supply chain with a different layout

Fig. 4. Diagram of the intralogistic process within the organization's supply chain with 4.0 technology

Table 3. Optimization characteristics in the study setting

	Warehouse	Distribution center
Principal function	Storage management and inventory layout	Flow management products
"Cost Driver" principal	Space and facilities	Transport, Hand working
Order cycle	Months, weeks	Days, hours
Activities of value-added	Punctual, in rotation Cyclical	They are an intrinsic part of process
Expeditions	On customer demand and Vendors	According to orders
Rotation of inventory	3, 6, 9, 12 - days	12, 24, 48, 96, 120 - days

Table 3 above are data obtained from the current scenario of the organization under study, where it is evident the application of concepts in the areas of process optimization, reengineering and distribution of plants for the full identification of the problem posed and the solution to it. As Jung puts it [24], "the new world scenario of globalization has made organizations transform, adapt and play new roles". In this way, international organizations and governments identified control strategies to mitigate the negative impact that can be generated in the process such as a new millennium project, created to discuss and evaluate the future challenges that humanity may have with 4.0 technologies [25].

3   Analysis of the Results Achieved and Statistical Evidence

The results of the instrument used are presented, and based on them, the solutions are presented according to the simulation model optimization used in each scenario the representation of the operations or activity of the logistics operators of the Colombian Caribbean region that are the object of this research study. The form of usability for the achievement of the results analyzed in this section is directed to the methodology exposed in the previous section, under the application of the proportional fixation criterion. However, the maintenance of statistical assumptions in the calculations is vital for the effectiveness of the inferences of this study. In the first subsection, a general description is presented on how the logistic operator selected for the present study has been found ahead of the component evaluated in the research. Next, it is established how are the relationships between the factors of the recommended scenarios and ends with impact analysis associated them, it is necessary to point out and identify the inferences derived from the data collected through an instrument with coherence, cohesion, reliability, and validity, which are indispensable elements in research activities:

i)   The Instrument: For this work, a reliable instrument is used to identify the organizational characteristics based on the horizontal and vertical analysis in the adaptation of 4.0 technologies, which allows defining the current situation of the organization and the future scenarios of analysis based on the information collected, which seeks to verify the absorption capacity of new technologies through the measurement quadrants, as well as the promotion and use of technology, giving present research project the base tool for the delimitation of the study factors of the model to be used. Determining the degree to which an instrument provides consistent and systematic data [26]. For the above, Cronbach's alpha is used to measure interior uniformity, to locate the results between the items based on the variances and correlations, for which the following formula should be applied:

$$\alpha = \left[\frac{k}{k-1}\right]\left[1 - \sum_{i=1}^{k}\frac{S_i^2}{S_t^2}\right]$$

Where: k is the number of reagents
$i = 1$: defines the index to which an initial value called the lower limit is assigned, in this case 1.
$S_i^2 =$ is the variance of each item.
$S_t^2 =$ is the variance of the instrument.
Reliability checks are carried out through the provision of measurement data instruments, prove their effectiveness in the field of logistics operators. For the purpose, the population to be studied is evaluated according to the characteristics of the logistics operators of the Colombian Caribbean region above 44 participants based on a critical analysis from the organization that is the subject of this study was selected to be a reference as a matrix in the adoption of the main characteristics in terms of adaptability to other organizations in the same environment. In the development analysis with the formula previously described, obtaining as a result $\alpha = 0.98$; affirming that its structure, based on the reliability criterion, is evaluated as excellent.

ii) Scenarios: They are defined as the development of the events that can occur or dissipate depending on the applicability of the simulation via optimization. For the present study, three scenarios are presented for the respective analysis and correlation with the feasibility of immersion of technologies 4.0 in the intralogistics activities of the logistics operator studied. For each scenario, the application of the factors that determine the evaluation of the organizational efficiency indexes is evidenced, developing the studied problem in each of the facets of the context with its distinctive results evidenced in Table 4, in which three aspects of mutual interest and determined in the analysis of the results of the vertical and horizontal integration systems are observed [23]:

- Supplier analysis: strengths, mutually beneficial relationships, communication, and integration between the organization under study and the organizations that supply the necessary inputs for the operation are evidenced.
- Organizational analysis: It establishes aspects inherent to the intralogistics activity within the organization and its improvement evaluations, with which it synthesizes the object of study of the research.
- Customer analysis: Observes the dependent and independent variables on which the requirements towards the product are based, according to the expectations

and needs of the customer; in this aspect the organizational efficiency indicator is established.

From the above, the Flexsim software as a working tool of the present research project allows to visualize the three study scenarios with the characteristics previously defined and allows to establish the conditions of decision making that impact on the improvement of organizational efficiency.

iii) Evaluation Method: The results obtained from the scenarios using the simulation model via optimization according to the tests of approval, integrity, and reliability of the simulation allow us to obtain the data evidenced in Table 4, which shows a comparison between the factors according to the indicators that interact for this study and how they fluctuate according to the scenario used, with the above it is established that the incorporation of 4.0 technologies is the necessary option to solve the problem posed and the objective of this research.
The table above shows the results obtained by simulating the scenarios established and parameterized in the statistical assumptions by the results of the previous analysis, which translates into obtaining information for decision making and the assumption as the solution to improve organizational efficiency, the objective of this study, focused on the adoption of 4.0 technology for the antiphlogistic processes of the logistics operators of the Colombian Caribbean region.

iv) Analysis of the research: It presents the analysis of the results obtained with the company object of study of the research about the diagnosis made, the analysis of the scenarios using the simulation model via optimization and the suggestions for the applicability of 4.0 technologies, to achieve higher levels of organizational efficiency. From the above, we can determine that the factors defined by the application of the instruments are directly related to the organizational efficiency index and taking into account the results detailed in Table 4 in the 4.0 technology scenario in relation to the scenarios of the current situation and different layout, it is determined that it is imperative to invest in the application of 4.0 technologies, which will allow the logistics operator under study to obtain a gradual and consistent improvement in its organizational efficiency. In addition, the following are established as analysis factors: Information Management and Business Model, Being the latter the one that is more favored of the use of the technologies 4.0 in the intralogistics activities of the logistic operators for the Colombian Caribbean region, which supposes an increase of the quality of the infrastructures until 90.45%. Likewise, it shows the level found in terms of implementation of technologies and the opportunities for new adaptations for them.

Similarly, Fig. 5 determines the application and result of the instrument that measures the capacity of the inclusion of 4.0 technologies in the company under study. Cronbach's Alpha coefficient is the most widely used indicator of the reliability of psychometric scales in the social sciences, which gives us a measure of the internal consistency of the reagents that make up a scale. If this measure is high, we assume that we have evidence of the homogeneity of the scale, i.e. that the items are "pointing" in the same direction, which is evidenced by the application of this measure to the results in Fig. 6. That is, we assume that our scale is Tau equivalent or essentially Tau equivalent. In conclusion,

Table 4. Table of analysis of the projected scenarios

Factors	Indicators	Scenarios		
		Current	Different distribution or layout	Technology 4.0
Information management	Volume of purchases	32.12%	30.59%	34.55%
	Inventory time	28.56%	36.45%	50.61%
Strategic planning	Perfect delivery received	36.54%	30.29%	44.37%
	Inventory time	28.78%	50.18%	58.85%
	Types of transport	22.54%	82.62%	59.93%
	Punctuality of the offices	30.23%	42.51%	73.17%
Subcontracting	Perfect delivery received	8.71%	14.63%	44.77%
Business model	Certificate of suppliers	54.38%	74.48%	84.49%
Logistic barriers	Quality of infrastructure	64.81%	80.07%	90.45%
Cost	Order quality	70.23%	58.15%	68.38%
	Perfect delivery received	36.19%	30.74%	44.02%
	Inventory time	28.70%	36.52%	38.27%
Risk	Volume of purchases	22.76%	38.38%	28.68%
	Efficiency in the offices customs officers	82.94%	86.17%	84.48%
Distribution strategy	Types of transport	8.67%	6.05%	11.33%
	Punctuality of the offices	40.42%	30.72%	44.57%

about the results, the instruments present a reliable and trustworthy data, which allows to characterize and observe the need that the logistic operator has as shown in Fig. 7 for the primordial factor that influences the cost variable, which is the angular point of the measurement of the organizational efficiency; therefore it is necessary that the company under study passes from quadrant 2 to 3 as shown in Fig. 5 for to the adaptation of the technologies of the industry 4.0, and consequently give solution to the problem studied in the present project.

Figure 5 shows the result of the application of the instrument of vertical and horizontal integration in the framework of industry 4.0; which is described as the diagnostic result of

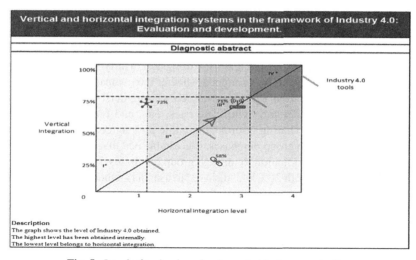

Fig. 5. Level of technology implemented in the organization

the organization under study, showing the reality of the environment studied, the ability to adopt new technologies and the level of absorption it has for it. The organization under study according to the results is in a very good quadrant of opportunity established between 71% to 75% of absorption which allows a good margin of improvement to continue growing in the adaptability of emerging technologies in terms of continuous improvement of its processes and indicators.

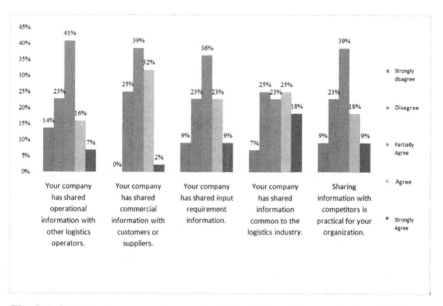

Fig. 6. Information management as a major factor in improving organizational efficiency

Figure 6 shows the results of the predominant factor in this study, Information Management, the result of the internal load generator instrument; with which it was obtained as a result for this factor for logistics operators under the indicators of purchase volume and inventory time, it was estimated that 41% disagreed. Thirty-nine percent strongly agreed with this strategy. Next, we examined whether the company shares operational and/or commercial information with its customers or suppliers, such as safety information, driver databases, delivery schedules, rates, etc., and found that 32% of the companies disagreed with sharing information, while 25% agreed with this option for their processes. To manage group purchases, it is established that 25% of the company partially agree to share information to manage group purchases, followed by 25% who agree and do so, together with 26% who disagree to use this method in their information and purchasing processes.

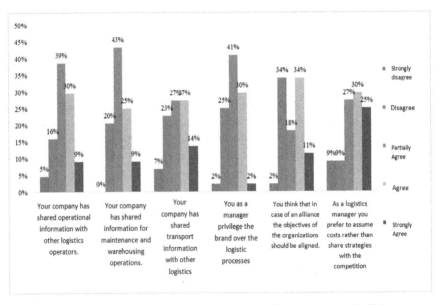

Fig. 7. Business model as a major factor in improving organizational efficiency

Figure 7 shows the results of the second predominant factor in the organization under study, the Business Model, which has a very dynamic system in the way it operationalizes its processes in terms of supply chain collaboration, in the search for increased organizational efficiency. In which it is observed that 39% of the company under study emphasizes to be partially in agreement in sharing resources, followed by 30% in agreement. We went on to examine whether the company has shared facilities for cross docking operations or for vehicle maintenance with other logistics operators, where 43% of the company highlighted that they partially agree and have done so, followed by 25% who confirmed that they agree with the strategy. The study continues to determine the participation in joint ventures by examining if the company has participated in joint ventures of transportation operations with other logistics operators, where it is obtained that 27%

of the company highlights to agree and have implemented it and 27% of the studied population indicates to be partially in agreement with the participation. The next question is whether the logistics manager gives priority to brand recall over the costs derived from not sharing some cargo operations with competitors. In this topic, the analysis is synthesized in privileging their brand over the costs derived, through the instrument it is determined that 45% of the companies consider to be partially in agreement, while 30% agree with the privilege of their brand. The analysis ends by asking whether the company thinks that in the case of a possible collaborative alliance, the business model of its company is incompatible with that of its competitors. It can be seen that 34% of the company agrees and has done so, followed by 34% who disagree.

4   Conclusions and Discussions of Information Analysis

The present study is framed in a quantitative research, under an epistemologically positivist approach, with which it is developed in the analysis of real facts evidenced by practice, identifying the main factors through the indicators that are used in the construction of scenarios on the application of simulation via optimization for the adoption of technologies 4.0 in the intralogistic activities towards the improvement of the efficiency indices of the logistic operators of the Colombian Caribbean region. The results obtained in this study validate trends correlated with information management factors and the business model as the central axis of the scenarios studied. The results achieved are defined as a far-reaching contribution to decision-making within the organizations of the Caribbean region concerning to logistics operators, likewise, the aim is to contribute to the state of knowledge through the influence exerted by the authors or theoreticians studied and evidenced in this research, who with their work allowed to give an orientation due to the analysis of information.

For the present study, a substantial improvement was obtained in the factors related to the organizational efficiency index, described in Table 4, where we can evidence a major increase between 4% and 11% per item studied. The operationalization of the factors, determine a series of aspects that allow evidencing the need to improve all the stages of the intralogistics process, in general terms the organization and its studied sector must identify that allow them to improve their decision making that influence the organizational efficiency. By the application of Industry 4.0 technologies in intralogistics processes in general terms: special attention should be paid to the variables of strategic planning and subcontracting, as these are the ones that gradually impact intralogistics costs.

References

1. Lambert, D.M., Cooper, M.C., Pagh, J.D.: Supply chain management: implementation issues and research opportunities. Int. J. Logist. Manage. **9**(2), 1–20 (1998). https://doi.org/10.1108/09574099810805807
2. DIAN: Dirección de Impuestos y Aduanas Nacionales. 07 July (2018). https://www.dian.gov.co/. Accessed 23 Oct 2019

3. Silva, J.D.: Gestión de la cadena de suministro: una revisión desde la logística y el medio ambiente. Entre Ciencia Ingeniería **11**(22), 51–59 (2017). http://www.scielo.org.co/scielo.php?script=sci_arttext&pid=S1909-83672017000200051&lng=en&tlng=es. Accessed 03 Nov 2020
4. Orjuela-Castro, J.A., Suárez-Camelo, N., Chinchilla-Ospina, Y.I.: Costos logísticos y metodologías para el costeo en cadenas de suministro: una revisión de la literatura. Cuadernos Contabilidad **17**(44), 377–420 (2016). https://dx.doi.org/10.11144/Javeriana.cc17-44.clmc
5. Johnson, M.P., Midgley, G., Chichirau, G.: Emerging trends and new frontiers in community operational research. Eur. J. Oper. Res. **268**(3), 1178–1191 (2018). https://doi.org/10.1016/j.ejor.2017.11.032
6. Mera, C.: UNAD. Retos y Desafíos de la Prospectiva en las Organizaciones del Futuro. Grupo de Investigación y Estudios Prospectivos y Estrategicos (2019). ISBN 978-958-651-600-6
7. Dornier, P.-P., Ernst, R., Fender, M., Kouvelis, P.: Global Operations and Logistics: Text and Cases. Hardcover (1998). Jan. 1 1714
8. i Cos, J.P., de Navascués, R., Gasca: Manual de logística integral. EdicionesDíaz de Santos, Madrid (2001). ISBN 84-7978-345-1
9. Roux, M.: Manual de logística para la gestión de almacenes. Gestión, Barcelona (2000, 2003). ISBN 10: 8480881720
10. Ballou, R.: Logística administración de la cadena de suministro. Pearson Educación, México (2004). ISBN 970-26-0540-7
11. Carranza, O., Sabria, F.: Logística: mejores prácticas en Latinoamérica. Internacional Thomson Editores, México (2005). ISBN13: 9789706864116
12. Christopher, M.: Logística aspectos estratégicos. Limusa, México (1999). ISBN 9789681852825
13. Casas, G.G., Romero, B.P.: Logística y distribución física: evolución, situación actual, análisis comparativo y tendencias. McGraw-Hill Interamericana, Madrid (1998). ISBN 84-481-1366-7
14. Smykay, E.W.: Physical Distribution Management: Logistics Problems of the Firm. A Macmillan Marketing Book. Macmillan, New York (1961). (OCoLC)614422824
15. Duran, S.: Liderazgo transformacional como estrategia de adaptación en la gestión logística empresarial. Rev. Desarrollo Geren. **4** (2017)
16. Farris, M.T.: Evolution of academic concerns with transportation and logistic. Transp. J. **37**, 42–50 (2017). https://www.jstor.org/stable/20713336
17. Chen, R., Liu, L., Wu, J.: Logistics capability and its grey assessment model. In: International Conference on IEEE Grey Systems and Intelligent Services (2007). https://doi.org/10.1109/GSIS.2007.4443455
18. Sanchez, O.: Guía para la construcción y análisis de indicadores. Departamento Nacional de Planeación. Bogota (2018)
19. Botthof, A.: Zukunft der arbeit im kontext von autonomik und industrie 4.0. In: Botthof, A., Hartmann, E.A. (eds.) Zukunft der Arbeit in Industrie 4.0, pp. 3–8. Springer, Heidelberg (2015). https://doi.org/10.1007/978-3-662-45915-7_1
20. BID: Logística Urbana: Los desafíos de la Distribución Urbana de Mercancías. Centro de Estudios Económicos para el Desarrollo y la Competitividad, Cámara de comercio de Cartagena (2009). https://publications.iadb.org/es/publicacion/14260/logistica-urbana-los-desafios-de-la-distribucion-urbana-de-mercancias
21. de Lima, P., Orlem, B.S., Sandro, R.T., Manuel, C., Follmann, N.: Una nueva definición de la logística interna y forma de evaluar la misma. Ingeniare Rev. Chilena Ingeniería **25**(2), 264–276 (2017). https://doi.org/10.4067/S0718-33052017000200264
22. La Rosa, V.: Resumén ejecutivo 2016–2019. Gobernación, Atlantico (2019)
23. Pérez: Sistemas de integración vertical y horizontal en el marco de industria 4.0: Evaluación y desarrollo. UANL, Monterrey (2017). http://eprints.uanl.mx/id/eprint/16246

24. Jung, K.: Mapping strategic goals and operational performance metrics for smart manufacturing systems. Proc. Comput. Sci. **44**, 184–193 (2015). https://doi.org/10.1016/j.procs.2015.03.051
25. Rennung, C.: Service Provision in the Framework of Industry 4.0. Proc.-Soc. Behav. Sci. **221**, 372–377 (2016). https://doi.org/10.1016/j.sbspro.2016.05.127
26. Hernandez Sampieri, F.: Metodología de la Investigación. McGraw Hill, México (2014). ISBN 978-607-15-0291-9
27. Mejía, L.: Documentos CONPES consejo nacional de política económica y social república de Colombia departamento nacional de planeación, Bógota (2018). https://colaboracion.dnp.gov.co/CDT/Conpes/Econ%C3%B3micos/3918.pdf
28. Orozco E.A.J.: Proyecto Pilito Corredor Logistico en Ultima Milla y Logistica Urbana en Barranquilla y su Area Metropolitana. Barranquilla: informegeneral al Ministerio de Transporte (2017)

Sustainability Model for the Livestock Sector in the Department of La Guajira - Colombia

Helia Rosa del Carmen Daza Guerra[✉], Carlos Jose Regalao-Noriega,
and Karen Acosta Triana

Facultad de Ingenierías, Universidad Simón Bolívar, Barranquilla, Atlantico, Colombia
{helia.daza,cregalao,karen.acosta}@unisimonbolivar.edu.co

Abstract. A sustainability model allows present needs to be met without compromising future needs. Based on this, this study shows the development of a sustainability model for the livestock sector in the Guajira department in Colombia, where an analysis is made of the most relevant factors of the business, the characteristics of the area, the livestock and how everything impacts on the development of the activity in the environment. The analysis is based on three relevant perspectives, namely the economic, social and environmental levels, which, through the methodology used, emphasize the three pillars of sustainability applied to livestock farming in order to transform the sector into an environment that is sustainable over time.

Therefore, this research seeks to provide solutions to the needs of the sector in the environment studied and to provide sustainable characteristics to the area of action of livestock in the Guajira - Colombia, trying to increase the efficiency of the sector in relation to its stakeholders.

Keywords: Livestock · Sustainability · Sustainable development

1 Introduction

Taking as an example advanced capitalist countries such as Canada, Australia and New Zealand, which have development models focused on the use of agricultural resources for the leverage of their economies, we find that Colombia, being a developing country with a great capacity to exploit these resources, has focused its development opportunities on models that ultimately leave the primary sector of the economy behind. At present, the livestock sector in our country represents 1.6% of the national GDP [1], a representative percentage taking into account that livestock farming is an individual and above all rural activity.

Cattle breeding continues to be very important for the socio-economic development of the country, representing 88% of the national agricultural area [2]. Livestock production generates income and provides employment opportunities, not only for producers, but also for different workers during the production and distribution of food of animal origin. Hundreds of millions of people living in rural areas keep livestock in traditional

J. A. Marmolejo-Saucedo et al. (Eds.): COMPSE 2021, LNICST 393, pp. 196–215, 2021.
https://doi.org/10.1007/978-3-030-87495-7_13

production systems, to ensure their livelihoods, as a safety net and to help meet household food needs [3].

Livestock farming is one of the main activities of the agro-industrial sector in Colombia, with a 3.6% growth in GDP in 2018 compared to 2017 [4], supplying the country with milk and meat. According to the Ministry of Agriculture and Rural Development, the share of livestock in agricultural GDP is 9.1%; however, according to FEDEGAN in 1925, agricultural GDP accounted for 57% of the country's total GDP. Today it only accounts for 6.3%. In 1950, cattle farming contributed 14% of the total GDP, and today it contributes 1.4% as shown in Fig. 1 [1].

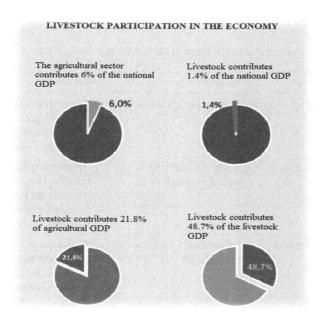

Fig. 1. Livestock participation in the Colombian economy. [Fedegan, 2018].

Livestock activity is present in 27 of Colombia's 32 departments, which means that a large number of the Colombian population is involved in this activity. For many years, it has been the way of life for peasants and businessmen in Colombia, and one of the main sources of income for the country, which is why it is of great importance in national agricultural and agro-industrial production [5]. This activity generates 810,000 direct jobs representing 6% of national employment and 19% of employment in agricultural activities [6]. In addition, Colombia has 26.2 million cattle, 597,177 cattle farms, 219 processing plants and a production of approximately 757,789 tons of meat in 2017, whose commercialization generated 7.2 billion for the country's economy. On the other hand, milk production is 7.1 billion litres per year and formal milk collection is 3.5 billion litres [1].

Colombia's livestock landscapes present a wide heterogeneity in terms of the ecosystems in which they are located and the arrangements used in cattle grazing areas [8]. Livestock farming in Colombia has evolved in the 20th century especially through improvements in breeds, pastures and nutrients. However, extensive cattle raising continues to predominate, as the main form of livestock exploitation within the highly heterogeneous structure [7]. Natural habitats include mature forests, secondary forests, thickets and riparian corridors, among others. Although traditionally treeless pasture has been used for cattle production, different types of silvopasture systems have been successfully established in the country in recent decades, contributing to improved sustainability and more efficient livestock production [8]. This is justified in each of the departmental development plans of the Colombian Caribbean region summarized in Table 1.

Table 1. Development plans department of La Guajira and municipalities. Own creation.

Plan De Desarrollo	Nombre	Retos
Departamento de La Guajira	"Unidos por el Cambio"	"Impulsar la tecnificación del sector agropecuario y el acceso a crédito y mercados nacionales e internacionales"
Municipio de San Juan del Cesar	"Es el momento del cambio para el progreso social"	"Implementación de Buenas Prácticas Ganaderas (BPG)." Acciones del Programa de Ganadería Colombiana Sostenible en el municipio
Municipio de Barrancas	"Historia de Cambio y Prosperidad"	"Fortalecer el sector pecuario en el municipio" "Realizar un programa de Ganadería Integral sostenible"(bovinos, porcinos, caprinos)
Municipio de El Molino	+ Oportunidades + Progreso	"Fortalecida la economía del municipio brindando apoyo técnico y tecnológico a las labores agropecuarias de la población campesina de la región
Municipio Fonseca	"Unidos Podemos"	"Apoyar a la implementación de prácticas agropecuarias productivas sostenibles de arroz y Ganadería"
Municipio Villanueva	"Villanueva de Todos"	"Desarrollo Económico agropecuario y turístico para todos"

(*continued*)

Table 1. (*continued*)

Plan De Desarrollo	Nombre	Retos
Municipio Urumita	"Construyamos lo nuestro", "Urumita Gana"	"Urumita fortalece al campo – sector agropecuario y agroindustrial"
Municipio Manaure	"Con EnfoqueÉtnicodiferencial"	"Plan integral, de corto, mediano y largo plazo, multisectoriales y multidisciplinarios para estimular y recuperar la actividad agropecuaria tecnificada y eficiente en el departamento", "Implementación de Buenas Prácticas Ganaderas"
Municipio Riohacha	"Cambia la historia"	"Mejorar las capacidades de los pequeños productores rurales para la inclusión y participación sostenible en las cadenas de valor agropecuarias"

The year 2018 was a difficult one for cattle farming because it had many ups and downs and the problem of the health crisis had a serious and dramatic impact on the economy of this agricultural sub-sector of the country. Similarly, it is important to highlight that the strong summers impact the sector, making access to food and water sources difficult according to FEDEGAN [1]. Another issue that directly affects the sector is cattle theft, which leaves annual losses of 400 billion, according to DICAR in 2017, more than 3000 cattle were stolen in Colombia. As well as the low competitiveness of the sector, where the availability of the country's resources is wasted [9].

Taking as a reference the whole context and the needs presented in the sector, this article proposes a sustainability model that goes in the direction of making the livestock activity sustainable in time, involving all the variables that intervene, in order to achieve an integral combination of economy, environmental and social management in the livestock farms. This is done by analyzing representative variables in each of the dimensions of economic, environmental and social sustainability, achieving the sustainability of the sector with the integration of these three elements. Sustainability is an issue that has been gaining strength as the years go by, taking such relevance due to climate change and the consequences it brings with it, so this analysis is required, on one of the sources of pollution. In this sense, the proposed model is aimed at waste reduction and utilization, equity and social integration, communication and understanding of the problems in the sector and good profitability.

1.1 Sustainability and the Livestock

The society of the 21st century requires the incorporation of sustainable development in its daily life [8], covering the three economic, social and environmental dimensions, in order to make the process integral. Several studies have identified that companies do not develop a sustainability strategy because it is not their priority, they do not have a good command of the subject and there is a dilemma between being sustainable or profitable [10]. Therefore, sustainability can be seen as a new approach within business, where companies seek to promote social inclusion, optimize natural resources and reduce environmental impact, without neglecting the economic and financial viability of the company.

Although the concept of sustainable development does not have a single definition. However, historians of the concept place its origins in the environmental movement and environmental economics [11], In livestock systems, the concept of sustainability was developed in the 1990s, and has undergone changes over the years due to the nature of these systems. On the one hand, we can observe more or less intensified livestock systems where essentially productivist objectives prevail and where the version of weak sustainability predominates. On the other hand, we can observe extensive and ecological systems, where the balance of the social, economic and environmental dimensions is evident and where the version of strong sustainability predominates [12].

The main objective of sustainability is to reconcile economic growth with care for the social environment and environmental protection. However, in an environment of uncertainty, companies need tools to help them make decisions and define their strategies. Therefore, in view of this new reality, it is necessary to consider the use of models that allow the rediscovery of new ways of managing not only companies but also their objectives, strategies and policies in order to make the prosperity of companies compatible with a sustainable quality of life at a planetary level. To this end, we must rely on flexible models that allow for the hybrid processing of objective data and subjective estimates, that make it possible to forecast the future behavior of companies, institutions and social agents, and that make it possible to offer a redesign in the economic relations that affect all the entities involved" [12].

The models of sustainability that have been developed throughout history in Latin America are based on three elements: economic growth, fiscal stability and economic integration. However, for the contemporary era, they have shown a relevant shift, covering aspects that go beyond the economic, including human development, autonomy, multidimensionality and environment. "Many of the interpretations of sustainable development agree that, in order to achieve this, policies and actions to achieve economic growth must respect the environment and also be socially equitable in order to achieve economic growth" [13]. In addition, Garzon and Mares [14] in their work they comment that "sustainability is a complex and multidimensional concept that cannot be solved by a single corporate action and companies are faced with the challenge of minimizing waste from ongoing operations, preventing pollution, together with the reorientation of their portfolio of skills towards more sustainable technologies and technologically clean skills".

Como objetivo principal del desarrollo sostenible es la creación del valor dentro del negocio o en el proceso, por medio de la actividad comercial, que se pueda lograr a través de la propia actividad comercial de la empresa, la disminución del consumo de electricidad, agua y otras materias primas, el uso de nuevas tecnologías y la innovación de productos [15].

In terms of Sustainable Livestock, Colombia has focused on a concept of integral sustainability, which includes Economic Sustainability, Environmental Sustainability and Social Sustainability. According to Celso Alfredo Salazar, 2011 "Livestock and agro-productive activities, in general, are under great pressure due to the changing competitive conditions that, in an increasingly dynamic and global scenario, require livestock producers to have skills that are not only productive, but also strategic in the search for markets and the generation of added value for their production. [16] In this sense, a strategy must be sought for improvement at the productive, environmental and social levels, focused on the sustainable development of the livestock sector.

1.2 Livestock in the Guajira

Specifically, the department of La Guajira occupies the 25th place in extension with 20,848 km^2 equivalent to 1.8% of the national territory, located in the area called "dry Caribbean". The region is characterized by three main productive activities such as mining and quarrying, and social, communal and personal service activities and the productive orientation of the livestock of La Guajira, is focused on breeding (50% of the herd) and the dual purpose (46%) as shown in Fig. 2 [1].

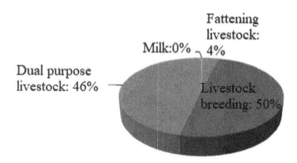

Fig. 2. Productive orientation of La Guajira. [Foro Ganadería Regional 2014–2018 Guajira.]

Its cattle inventory is one of the smallest in the country, occupying 20th place, with 330,000 cattle distributed in 4,591 farms, occupying an area of 1,578,371 ha. This characterises the Guajira's cattle ranch as one of the lowest in terms of load capacity (0.22 head/ha). Guajira cattle ranching produces 389 million litres of milk per year (1,066,000 L of milk per day) 10, and slaughters around 520,000 cattle (2013), according to the Fedegan established in the Regional Livestock Forum [1]. The department has 15 municipalities distributed in 3 sub-regions: Guajira Alta (Uribía and Manaure), Guajira Media (Riohacha, Maicao, Dibulla and Albania) and Guajira Baja (Hatonuevo, Barrancas, Fonseca, Distracción, San Juan del Cesar, El Molino, Villanueva, Urumita and La Jagua del Pilar), the activity is concentrated in the lower Guajira.

Similarly, the department of La Guajira is affected year after year by factors such as low competitiveness (production and application of new technologies), climate change, theft of livestock and outlaw groups, health problems (foot and mouth disease). In general, there are many advantages in favors of production such as access to water, availability of pasture and feed, having a large herd and adequate agro-ecological conditions. However, there are deficiencies in the competitive advantages in milk and meat production, given that the use of good technologies and processes that lead to efficient indicators compared to international standards.

One of the points that most affects the productivity of the sector is climate change, where you can find very dry summers or wetter winters. According to the Fedegan [1], Between 2009 and 2012 there were two La Niña phenomena, and an El Niño phenomenon, causing the displacement of 2 million cattle and the death of more than 180,000. Given that the department of La Guajira is located in the dry Caribbean of Colombia, it is one of the sectors most affected by climate change, bringing as a consequence for the farms a lower availability of water for irrigation and watering holes for the cattle, the increase in production costs in terms of the use of labor to feed the cattle, the purchase of food inputs, vitamins and inject able tonics, a higher incidence of forest fires and the deterioration of the pastures. Likewise, for the animals there is a loss of weight due to dehydration, an increase in parasite problems and diseases (tick fever, diarrhea and pneumonia); due to a decrease in fodder consumption and caloric and water stress, there is a decrease in milk and meat production, and in the birth rate [17]. In accordance with all the previous problems, the identification of the variables involved in the sustainability of the sector and the existence of a validated model that allows this sustainability to be achieved, and the redesign of the livestock activity, seeking to ensure that all the points that directly affect the sector, such as climate change, the lack of technology, the fact that it is an uncompetitive sector, the groups on the margins of the law, among others, can reduce their impact and make the livestock sector in the department sustainable over time.

Since livestock farming is one of the most relevant activities in the Colombian economy, it is necessary to focus on seeking improvements in the sector and to have a prospective view of Colombian livestock farming for the coming years; this is in order to avoid the different variables impacting the sector, having a vision and projection of the business. Nowadays, cattle breeders must improve their productivity and competitiveness within the farm, in order to have international standards that allow us to compete in the foreign market; therefore, it is of vital importance to define efficient productive models. Likewise, it is necessary to demand the adequate conditions for competitiveness such as interest rates, development of roads and infrastructure, cost policy among others, greater state support for the rural sector, clear public policies towards agriculture and strong institutions; and in this way better manage the serious market problems that affect this sector.

2   Materials and Methods

As detailed in Fig. 3, the methodological approach on which the research is based is of a mixed type; quantitative and qualitative data will be collected, analyzed and interpreted in order to obtain answers to the problem posed and to help with the analysis of the descriptive context of the livestock sector. Therefore, a review of the literature will be carried out in order to obtain all the information related to the development of the sustainability model, and as an important part of the development of the model, the administrative methodology of each farm will be analyzed through surveys to farmers and employees, in order to obtain details of the farm management, to analyze the specific characteristics of the business. With the above, a content analysis was conducted, involving literary analysis and primary sources of information with which the variables were defined and the development of the model was carried out.

As detailed in Fig. 3, the methodological approach underpinning the research is a mixed one. Quantitative and qualitative data collection, analysis and interpretation will be carried out in order to obtain answers to the problem posed and will assist with the analysis of the descriptive context of the livestock sector. The administrative methodology of each farm will also be analyzed through surveys of farmers and employees, in order to obtain details of farm management, to analyze the specific characteristics of the business.

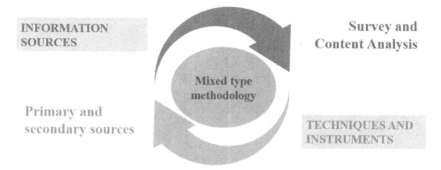

Fig. 3. Materials y methods. Own creation.

2.1 Source of Information

For the development of the investigation they are the primary and secondary sources, where testimonies and information of the stakeholders who intervene in the process will be gathered by means of a survey. In the same way secondary sources will be taken into account like statistics of the DANE, ICA among others, in order to obtain a wider information of the characteristics of the sector.

2.2 Techniques and Instruments

As an important part of the research process, direct information will be sought from farmers, workers and in general from all the relevant stakeholders in the project, with which relevant information will be taken, with which improvements can be defined and projected for the sector. Similarly, through the analysis of content, a subsequent study of the information collected in the surveys is carried out, also with secondary information from entities such as Fedegan, MinAgriculture, ICA, among others.

2.3 Procedure

Three stages are taken into account for the development of the project, detailed in Fig. 4, which begin with the collection of data, primary sources through a survey. Secondary sources are also analysed, including a literature review and statistics on the sector provided by government agencies. From this point onwards, we proceed to triangulate the dimensions of sustainability and the variables involved in the livestock process, building the model. The final stage is the validation of the model, where the type of validation methodology is established, to then proceed with the validation of the model.

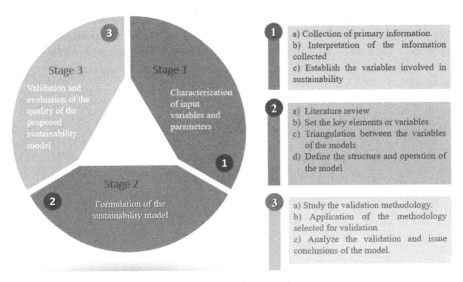

Fig. 4. Process. Own creation

3 Results

3.1 Defined Variables

Given the situation of livestock farming in the department of La Guajira, the following variables are defined for the model, focusing the sector on sustainability, with three dimensions, focusing on the triple bottom line, for the development of the model, where the economic, social and environmental dimensions are related as the main factors, and framing different variables that allow the sector to be analyzed from these, detailed in Table 2.

Table 2. Sustainability model factors and variables. Own creation.

Factores		Descripción	Variables	Descripción
Sustainability	Economic	Focused on the production of the good or the service, guaranteeing the development of the activity and the generation of profit by it	Productive areas	Large spaces where a wide variety of activities are developed for the creation or treatment of products
			Infrastructure	Necessary facilities for the development of an activity
			Technical and administrative records	Consignment of relevant data in a document; being evidence of the information official form
			Additional expenses in summer	Incurred expenses that complement the 'main expense' incurred
	Social	It is based on principles focused on creating just social conditions	Health, safety and well-being in workers	Focused on the prevention of occupational injuries and illnesses, in addition to the protection and promotion of workers' health
			Biosecurity	Norms, protocols, and principles to avoid risk to health and the environment from biological agents

(*continued*)

Table 2. (*continued*)

Factores		Descripción	Variables	Descripción
	Enviromental	Use natural resources responsibly, bearing in mind that it is not possible to replace natural capital	Environmental management	Plan for the prevention, mitigation, control, compensation and correction of negative environmental effects or impacts, given by the development of an activity
			Animal welfare and treatment	State in which the animal is found, taking into account the living conditions appropriate to its needs
Ganadería	Economic	Focused on the profitability of the business, seeking to be a productive farm throughout the year	Productive areas	Type of activities carried out within the farm in addition to livestock
			Infrastructure	The farm must have the necessary infrastructure for the livestock activity to develop fully
			Additional expenses in summer	Given the arid area where the activity takes place, additional food expenses are incurred due to the low production of natural grass on the farm

(*continued*)

Table 2. (*continued*)

Factores		Descripción	Variables	Descripción
	Social	Stable and fair conditions for workers and the community	Health, safety and well-being in workers	Trained personnel, affiliated with the EPS and ARL, the house has the necessary resources to live with dignity
			Biosecurity	Development of activities for the conservation and security of the environment where the activity takes place, including biosafety equipment, disinfection programs, entry of authorized personnel on the farm, among others
	Ambiental	Minimize the environmental impact within the farm, in addition to animal care and welfare	Environmental management	Environmental activities are carried out on the farm that promote the correct use of the land and the farm's environment in general
			Animal welfare and treatment	Preventive diagnostic activities for farm animals, with medicines approved by the ICA

3.2 Definition of Steakholders

Within the livestock process, different stakeholders are involved, whether they are internal or external to the farm, and these stakeholders can directly or indirectly affect the process. In this case, stakeholders are included in the process in order to involve them in the model, highlighting the relationship between each dimension, the defined variables and the stakeholders. In Table 3, the stakeholders involved in the livestock process are shown:

Table 3. Stakeholder. Own creation

Partes Interesadas	Definición
Clients	Wholesale - Retailers
Farmer	Farm Owner
Employee	Managed - Farm Foreman
Investor	Investment in livestock
ICA	Colombian Agricultural Institute
Fedegan	Colombian Federation of Livestock
MinAgricultura	Department of agriculture
Comunity	Community that intervenes or is affected in the process
Providers	Food, services, etc. providers
Asocebú	Cebuino Cattle Association
Other Livestock Farms	Alliances with other farms
Financial entities	Capital for investment

Stakeholders include customers, wholesalers and retailers, including the type of product to be purchased, either milk or meat, farmers as owners of the company, employees, investors in livestock, government entities, suppliers of inputs needed for the process, grass, seeds, associations such as Asocebu, alliances with other farms, financial institutions. In general, they intervene in the livestock as a fundamental part, for the development of the process, leading to the final objective of the farm, either for meat production, milk, or dual purpose.

3.3 Selection of the Sustainability Model for the Livestock Sector

The study carried out by Juan Plasencia et al. shows that the most referenced and implemented sustainable development models are TBL and the four-pillar model. These models are the basis for most of the instruments, standards, indices and indicators developed by international organizations and institutions. [18] According to the theory of sustainability different variations can be found which can be seen in Table 4.

Bearing in mind that the TBL model is one of the most used at present, and that it can be perfectly adjusted to the livestock sector, in order to seek sustainability based on the three economic dimensions, in search of utility and constant production during the year, social, taking into account that most of the employees in the sector belong to vulnerable groups and with respect to the generation of employment in society and the environment, focused on the welfare and treatment of animals and the preservation of the environment, as an important part within the process of the development of the activity. Similarly, this model of sustainability has some variations depending on the relationship and importance of the dimensions.

– Dimensions as independent systems

Table 4. Theoretical models of sustainability. Own creation.

Tipos De Modelos De Sostenibilidad		
Triple bottom line	TBL o 3BL	Sustainable development must be evaluated from three dimensions, economic benefits, achievements in equity and social justice and protection of the environment
Pressure - state - response and variations	PER	The impact that human activities exert on the environment, results in changes in the quality and quantity of environmental conditions (state), or what society responds through through environmental, economic and social actions
4 pillars of sustainability		The CDS, I call the four pillars of sustainability: economic, social, environmental and institutional
Lowell center for sustainable production	LSCP	A new model based on environmental, safety and health aspects of production
Sustainable balanced scorecard	SBSC	Its objective is to incorporate ecological, social and ethical aspects to the strategic core of the organization, through the balanced scorecard tool
Environment - social - governance model	ASG	It integrates the environmental, social and government dimensions. Used primarily for investment analysis
Cubrix model	Cubrix	It proposes the development of seven key levels in the management of the organization

- The three dimensions are related to each other
- The three dimensions are equally important
- Ecological Dimension is the focus
- Economic dimension is the focus

For this case the model is selected where the three dimensions are related to each other, giving it the same relevance and showing the following economic-social, environmental-social and environmental-economic interactions.

3.4 Definition of the Sustainability Model

The main objective in a sustainable business is the creation of value. Achieving this through commercial activity, in the case of a livestock company, focused on reducing environmental impact, the use of new technologies, product innovation. All of which generates a greater profitability and impact on the needs of consumers measured through indicators. These are defined as aspects of interest to the company and are analysed on the basis of general corporate sustainability guidelines [15].

There are many factors involved in livestock systems that make them very complex, such as physical, sociological, economic, political factors, etc. These include and condition the production playing an important role in the evolution of the system. Many studies consider livestock systems as dynamic systems where the interrelation of the elements that make up the system generates a complexity inherent to its own nature that conditions the different production practices; location, demography, markets and production potential play an important role in the way these systems can evolve [12]. Livestock are generally raised mainly on grass, grazing land and non-food biomass from maize. millet, rice and sorghum crops and in turn provide manure and traction for future crops.

Animals act as insurance against hard times and provide farmers with a regular source of income from sales of milk, eggs and other products. Thus, in the face of population growth and climate change, smallholder farmers should be the first target of policies to intensify production - carefully managed inputs of fertilizer, water and feed to minimize waste and impact, supported by improved access to markets, new varieties and technologies [19]. A model of sustainability includes three very important aspects, economic, environmental and social; knowing the most relevant characteristics and problems in the sector, the following model is designed with the aim of having the sector become more sustainable by seeking an improvement in the supply of meat and milk products, being constant throughout the year, likewise focus the sector in favor of environmental conservation, waste reduction, the use of renewable energy, preserving native species and in the social sphere, the search for equity, support to the community, being fair with the remuneration of employees.

Economical: Improving the economy in the sector is one of the key and relevant points, taking into account the problems that arise in the Guajira, which prevent excellent results from being obtained. It is important to take into account good livestock practices, as well as to implement strategies that provide support to the livestock during the hardest time of the year and mitigate the consequences of summer in the sector, managing to keep the livestock in good condition, without lowering production and without incurring additional costs.

Environmental: In general, within the cattle company there are many environmental factors among which it is important to take into account, taking into account these are in the natural environment, in search of obtaining the resources of nature for animal welfare. Therefore, the management within the company must be focused towards the care of the environment, mitigating the impact that the activity may cause, as well as the animal welfare, as the main product.

Social: The sustainability model for the social aspect focuses on the generation of employment in the community, support for vulnerable groups, fair remuneration for employees, and optimization of the waste generated in the activity in order to generate an additional source of income for the community. In accordance with the definitions of sustainability and related dimensions, integrating the concept of livestock farming in the Guajira, the following general model is established in Fig. 5, where the relationship between the economic-social, economic-environmental and social-environmental dimensions can be seen, and in its integration, achieving sustainability in the sector.

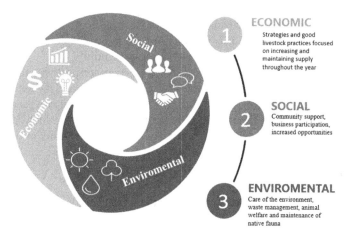

Fig. 5. General sustainability model. Own creation.

In accordance with the above, the sustainability model is defined by relating the variables, dimensions and related Stakeholders in the process and establishing the model involving the variables defined in Fig. 6.

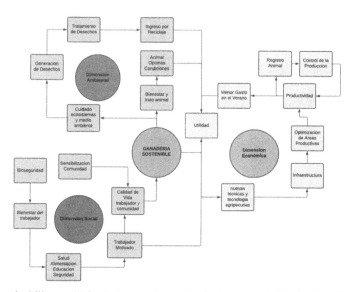

Fig. 6. Sustainability model for the livestock sector in the department of La Guajira. Own creation.

As shown in the image above, the variables defined above are involved, aiming at production, which would bring the livestock sector closer to sustainability.

- Economic Dimension: focused on improving investment in technology, improving infrastructure, optimizing the process, which helps to increase the utility of the farm.
- Social Dimension: aimed at two important parts, such as the welfare of the worker and biosecurity. From the above, it is possible to have motivated employees, positively impacting productivity, which helps us to increase the utility.
- Environmental Dimension: this is analyzed from two perspectives, the generation of waste and the well-being and treatment of animals; therefore, the aim is to obtain additional income with the treatment of the waste produced on the farm, and in addition to this, the maintenance of the livestock in optimum conditions, which contributes to the quality of the product generated, positively impacting the utility of the process.

3.5 Model Validation

The methodology selected for the validation of the sustainability model is Max Black's theory of models and metaphors [20]. In this way, taking into account the TBL sustainability model, it is projected towards the sustainability model of the livestock sector, focused on the most relevant variables that influence the development of the sector. In this sense, the structure of sustainable development can be seen in Fig. 7.

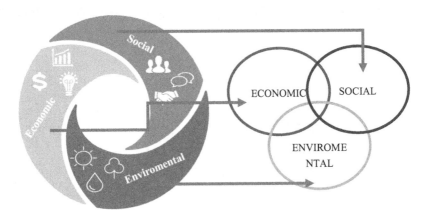

Fig. 7. Livestock sector model vs TBL model sustainable development.

The theory of Models and Metaphors proposed by Max Black, exposes the interaction of two object domains, each one containing a set of associated ideas that characterize and identify them. In this sense, the theoretical model of sustainability presented by John Elkington and the model proposed on the basis of this for the livestock sector in the department of La Guajira are analyzed, transferring the analysis of the three economic, social and environmental dimensions in the search for sustainability. Consequently, and following the guidelines of the theory of models and metaphors, the theoretical model interacts with the practical model for the livestock sector, where each of these has its associated ideas. In this way, the metaphor juxtaposes and transfers from a primary model the ideas and implications to the secondary model, illuminating certain features and obscuring others. The primary (theoretical) model is then seen through the framework of the secondary (practical) model. As a result it can be seen that the model planted on the basis of the theoretical one can be analysed that the two systems are seen as more similar to each other. In this sense, the interaction "creates" the similarities between the compared models. Given the application of the theory of the metaphor in the theoretical sustainability model towards the sustainability model of the livestock sector, finding the similarities, taking into account that the developed model is focused towards the theory of sustainability TBL, therefore, it can be said that the proposed model has a theoretical support, validating its content, given the translation of the plan-tee theory.

4 Discussion and Conclusions

In accordance with the established methodology and procedure, a sustainability model is defined for the department of La Guajira, framed by the characteristics of the sector, the stakeholders, the dimensions of sustainability, and the existing theoretical sustainability models. As a first step in the development of the project with the investigation of secondary sources, there are not many sources of information available regarding the subject under study. This led to the analysis of sustainability models from different sectors and different countries, with the aim of finding a reference as a guide, clarifying the form of the model, integrating it with the variables defined through the survey and different studies of the sector carried out in the department of La Guajira. The analysis of the livestock sector and the literature research led to the development of the model towards the triple bottom line (TBL), involving three dimensions, economic - social - environmental, which would lead the livestock sector of La Guajira to be sustainable over time. This is one of the most widely used models today, easily adjustable to the characteristics of the sector, including the relationship between the three dimensions, so that by complying with the model's guidelines, the sector can achieve sustainability.

In this way, each dimension or factor is related to the variables analyzed, the productive areas, technology, infrastructure, animal treatment and welfare, waste management, bio-security and worker welfare, focusing the processes within the farm on sustainable development. These variables frame the three dimensions, relating them to each other, which defines that the greater the focus of the farm on these three pillars, the greater the sustainability within it. Once the model had been defined, it entered the process of validation, but in the first instance, the different validation methods were analyzed, taking Max Black's theory of models and metaphors as a methodology. The author explains that it is possible to analyze the relationship between the theoretical model (Triple bottom line), and the practical model (Livestock sector in the Department of La Guajira), juxtaposing the characteristics of each one, and finding the similarities, managing to show that the practical model has the theoretical support. From the above, it is hoped that the sustainability model can frame a change in the sector, taking into account all the disadvantages that arise in the development of this, focused on the search for results in the economic dimension, with the increase in profits per year, reducing environmental impact and animal welfare, and in the social dimension, with the welfare of workers and biosecurity.

For the development of the model that adjusts to the characteristics and needs of the region, there is the inconvenience of the availability of information and literature, there are few works of sustainability models in the studied area, however, the theory of sustainability models is clear, so it can be easily transferred to a particular sector. Likewise, the study and analysis of the sector, taking primary sources as an important basis within the characterization of the model, identifying the relevant variables within it.

From the above, it is expected that the sustainability model can frame a change in the sector, taking into account all the problems that arise in its development, focused on the search for results in the economic dimension, with the increase of profits per year, the decrease of environmental impact and animal welfare, and in the social dimension, with the welfare of workers and biosafety. With the development of the sustainability model, it is expected to promote within the sector and in a region where conditions are becoming more unfavorable for the sector every year, with the impact of climate change, inequality, low product prices, which are making the sector less competitive and sustainable every day. In this sense, the analysis carried out provides the variables and conditions within the sector that allow livestock farming to be sustainable over time.

Likewise, in order to give continuity to the research, the need for the implementation of the model within a farm in the area is left open, in order to obtain accurate data and validation in real time of the model, obtaining information related to the variables and each dimension, leading to the analysis of new variables that were not contemplated in the model and that can be framed in the sustainable development of the sector. As well as the need to analyze the existing relationship between the model and the other regions of the Colombian Caribbean, making the comparison of the characteristics of each region and the applicability of the model within each department.

References

1. FEDEGAN: Foro ganadería regional visión 2014–2018 (2014)
2. Mahecha, L., Gallego, L., Peláez, F.: Situación actual de la ganadería de carne en Colombia y alternativas para impulsar su competitividad y sostenibilidad. Rev. Colomb. Ciencias Pecu. **15**(2), 213–225 (2002)
3. Makkar, H.P.S.: Aumento sostenible de la productividad del ganado mediante la utilización eficiente de los recursos alimenticios en países en vías de desarrollo, pp. 55–59 (2014)
4. DANE: Boletín Técnico Producto Interno Bruto (PIB) 2018, pp. 1–45 (2019)
5. ABC del Finkero: El problema de la ganadería en Colombia - ABC del Finkero (2013). http://abc.finkeros.com/el-problema-de-la-ganaderia-en-colombia/. Accessed 04 Nov 2019
6. Portafolio: La ganadería sigue siendo la actividad que más aporta al PIB I Economía I Portafolio (2017). https://www.portafolio.co/economia/la-ganaderia-sigue-siendo-la-actividad-que-mas-aporta-al-pib-509081. Accessed 04 Nov 2019
7. Cuenca, N., Chavarro, F., Díaz, O.: El Sector De Ganadería Bovina En Colombia. Aplicación De Modelos De Series De Tiempo Al Inventario Ganadero. Revista de. Rev. la Fac. Ciencias Econ. **16**(1), 165–177 (2008)
8. Nieto, J.A.M., Echeverri, C.G., Vega, C.J.Q., Chara, J., Medina, C.A.: Dung beetles associated with sustainable cattle ranching systems in different regions of Colombia. Biota Colomb. **21**(2), 134–141 (2020). https://doi.org/10.21068/C2020.V21N02A09

9. Ganadero, C.: DICAR reveló que en 2017 fueron hurtados 3.000 bovinos | CONtexto ganadero | Noticias principales sobre ganadería y agricultura en Colombia. https://www.contextogana dero.com/regiones/dicar-revelo-que-en-2017-fueron-hurtados-3000-bovinos. Accessed 04 Nov 2019

10. Carro Suárez, J., Reyes Guerra, B., Rosano Ortega, G., Garnica González, J., Pérez Armendáriz, B.: Modelo de desarrollo sustentable para la industria de recubrimientos cerámicos. Rev. Int. Contam. Ambient. **33**(1), 131–139 (2017). https://doi.org/10.20937/RICA.2017. 33.01.12

11. Chavarro, D., Vélez, M., Tovar, G., Montenegro, I., Hernández, A., Olaya, A.: Los Objetivos de Desarrollo Sostenible en Colombia y el aporte de la ciencia, la tecnología y la innovación. Colciencias **1**(3), 183–188 (2017)   .

12. Angón, E., García, A., Perea, J.: Evaluación de la sostenibilidad en sistemas ganaderos. Ambienta (118), 82–89 (2016). http://www.revistaambienta.es/WebAmbienta/marm/Dinami cas/secciones/articulos/Angon.htm

13. Miren, A.: Teoría de las Tres Dimensiones de Desarrollo Sostenible. Ecosistemas **2** (2002). https://doi.org/10.7818/RE.2014.11-2.00

14. Garzon, M., Mares, A.I.: Revisión Sobre la Sostenibildad Empresarial. Rev. Estud. Av. Liderazgo **1**, 52–77 (2018). https://www.regent.edu/acad/global/publications/real/vol1no3/4-cas trillon.pdf

15. Valencia-Rodríguez, O., Olivar-Tost, G., Redondo, J.M.: Modeling a productive system incorporating elements of business sustainability. DYNA **85**(207), 113–122 (2018). https://doi.org/ 10.15446/dyna.v85n207.71209

16. Salazar, C.A.: MERCADOS GANADEROS DE ALTO VALOR AGREGADO como alternativa comercial, no. 00086 (2011). http://www.sac.org.co/images/contenidos/Cartillas/Car tillaMercadosGanaderos.pdf

17. DANE: El fenómeno El Niño y sus efectos en la ganadería bovina colombiana. Boletín Mens. INSUMOS Y FACTORES Asoc. A LA Prod. Agropecu **24** (2014)

18. Antonio, J., Soler, P.: Modelos para evaluar la sostenibilidad de las organizaciones **34**(146), 63–73 (2018)

19. Herrero, M., et al.: Smart investments in sustainable food production: revisiting mixed crop-livestock systems. Science (80-) **327**(5967), 822–825 (2010). https://doi.org/10.1126/science. 1183725

20. Max, B.: Black_Max_Modelos_Y_Metaforas_pdf.pdf

Design of a Logistics Network Using Analytical Techniques and Agent-Based Simulation

Jose Antonio Marmolejo-Saucedo[1]([✉]) [iD], Roman Rodriguez-Aguilar[2] [iD],
Gerardo Meza Callejas[1,2] [iD], Mitchell Santiago Kelley Urbieta[1],
Saul Fernando Peregrina Acasuso[1] [iD], and Juan Pablo Gutierrez Girault[1] [iD]

[1] Facultad de Ingenieria, Universidad Panamericana, Augusto Rodin 498,
03920 Ciudad de Mexico, Mexico
jmarmolejo@up.edu.mx
[2] Facultad de Ciencias Economicas y Empresariales, Universidad Panamericana,
Augusto Rodin 498, 03920 Ciudad de Mexico, Mexico
rrodrigueza@up.edu.mx

Abstract. Business Logistics, or Supply Chain, has acquired a notorious relevance in current business management, due to its highly significant impact on the success of the production and service sectors. This work proposes the design of a supply chain that considers disruptive scenarios and improves the level of service compared to the current situation. Discrete event simulation techniques are used in conjunction with agent-based modeling to define production orders. A hypothetical case study was developed to show the performance of the proposal.

Keywords: Discrete event simulation · Supply chain design · Agent-based simulation

1 Introduction and Literature Review

Logistics network design in organizations helps define or validate the location, capacity, optimal number of nodes (plants, primary and secondary distribution centers, and cross-docking centers) and the flows between these nodes. The objective is to minimize the total cost of the network (production, transport, handling) and achieve the required service levels.

The supply chain is the sequence of suppliers that contribute to the creation and delivery of a merchandise or service to an end customer. Many processes and flows are involved within and outside of each link. Designing the most efficient supply chain for a business is a complex task, requiring planning for multiple variables. There are no magic solutions or models that work for any business. It

Supported by Universidad Panamericana.

J. A. Marmolejo-Saucedo et al. (Eds.): COMPSE 2021, LNICST 393, pp. 216–224, 2021.
https://doi.org/10.1007/978-3-030-87495-7_14

is necessary to know the characteristics of your company, its products and customers to create an optimal distribution chain. For example, in the pharmaceutical industry, which is one of the most complex supply chains, the combination of processes, operations and organizations involved in drug development and production is the perfect definition for the pharmaceutical industry [5]. Supply Chain problems often include both strategic and tactical decisions [3]. A characteristic of pharmaceutical companies is that the value of their inventory is of high value. This is to ensure a high level of customer satisfaction in the face of any operational disruption and to take advantage of any opportunities that arise (for example, increased demand during a disease outbreak). However, expensive inventories freeze capital and are undesirable for many reasons [7]. In practice, a periodic review inventory policy is not applicable for healthcare inventory management because customer demands and patient arrivals are uncertain. Therefore, efficient management of healthcare inventory systems requires a different approach than a periodic review order point model [8].

The mutual effects of the location of the facilities are related to inventory control decisions increasing the perishable factor. Product perishability is another critical problem in supply chains. Expired items can be overlooked and dispensed to patients, which could have potentially disastrous effects on both patient care as well as the reputation of the company [8]. Although designing an optimal supply chain becomes more complex when using perishable goods, few models take that factor into account [2]. In this study, the effects of opening a new production plant will be analyzed taking into account the location, management and handling of inventories, and cold chain distribution. You must take special care in inventory decisions that are made to ensure 100% product availability at the right time, at the right cost, and in good condition for customers. This will be done taking into account the inventory for a multiple product, a multiple period and a distribution network. Due to the dynamic and imprecise nature of the quantity and quality of the products manufactured. In a pharmaceutical industry supply chain, there is a high degree of uncertainty in the data when it is designed [4].

Therefore, in order to simulate various scenarios and see their effects, the model will be implemented in specialized software. Additionally, it is important to emphasize that we can generate profits taking in consideration the optimization of costs and make a green Supply Chain regulating CO_2 emission mainly with the transportation and distribution using methods like Center of Gravity and linear programming to establish the optimal location concentrating on Supply Chain sustainability. This impact will develop new opportunities based on protect the environment caused by the emissions of greenhouse gases (GHGs) and make more profits without the need to affect the environment.

Taking into account that an epidemic out-brake work in a similar way to a supply chain, some researchers address on how the simulation can help to predict the impact of this supply chain. Their studies are based on a global supply chain which includes multistage-suppliers, factory distribution center and customers in different continents. The models takes in consideration some assumptions, and some real facts, like the dates when the pandemic could have started. Taking into account three risks that make this type of supply chain special: long-term disruption existence and its unpredictable scaling, simultaneous disruption propagation and epidemic outbreak propagation and simultaneous disturbances in supply, logistics infrastructure and demand.

The methodology used to design the supply chain for a hypothetical case is presented below. We use discrete event simulation techniques to model the product flow in the network. Customer orders are modeled through agent-based simulation and the overall chain design is implemented in AnyLogistix software.

2   Methodology

The proposal considers a mathematical model to optimize product transport between the facilities that make up the logistics network. To verify the behavior of the model variables in the supply chain, a multi-paradigm simulation model is developed. This simulation model allows the parameters of the system to be varied dynamically in simulation time, it also allows describing and studying the impact of these changes. It is important to note that the simulation does not produce optimal solutions but rather describes the performance of the modeled system. After studying the performance of the system, it is possible to modify the structure of said system as well as the input parameters in order to optimize the overall performance versus the initial situation. In the design of the supply chain, the simulation carried out allows to optimize the configuration of the elements of the network, and suggests which and how many elements should be considered to make up the chain. The more details you consider, the more opportunities you have to find improvements. In companies, a very important factor is the planning of facilities and investments in equipment, material and physical spaces. The success of the operation of the company will depend on this planning. The software used allows us to implement the simulation proposal to identify the optimal locations to serve current and potential clients. Where more people live, the demand for the products is more likely, see Fig. 1.

In this work, this tool will be used and another location for a new plant will be proposed using a Greenfield Analysis (GFA). The software uses real terrain lines allowing a more exact optimal location solution. This resolution part takes into account the location of customers, products, demand for product and distance between customers, distribution centers and plants. For the study of the various alternatives, the different proposals (operating scenarios) must be simulated. These operating alternatives consider a different number of customers and their demands as well as the number and quantity of production orders. The alternatives considered are:

- Scenario 1A.- Optimal location GFA
- Scenario 2A.- Optimal location with + 30% demand
- Scenario 3A.- Optimal location with + 100% demand

Scenarios 1A only take into account current situation (demand). With this assumption, an increase in customers is not considered.

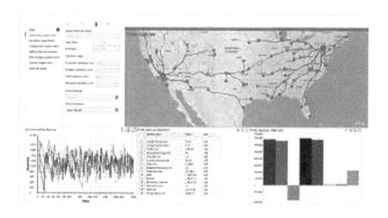

Fig. 1. AnyLogistix software

3   Mathematical Model

The proposed simulation model uses a mathematical model that optimizes the location of new facilities, for example factories and distribution centers. These facilities consider the locations of current customers and the quantity they demand. This optimization process is based on mathematical models of location called center of gravity models. The information that feeds these models is the following, see Fig. 2 and Fig. 3.

Greenfield Analysis is performed by solving a location model called Center of Gravity.

$$C_x = \frac{\sum_i d_{ix} w_i}{\sum_i w_i} \tag{1}$$

$$C_y = \frac{\sum_i d_{iy} w_i}{\sum_i w_i} \tag{2}$$

Where:
$d_i x = x$ coordinate of the locality i
$d_i y = y$ coordinate of the locality i
$w_i =$ volumen for the locality i

The software used allows to geographically locate the points in space, which makes the proposals obtained consider real paths between the facilities, that is, no Euclidean or straight solutions are proposed. Therefore, it is an advantage that we have if we only use classic mathematical programming models [6].

CLIENTS	X	Y	PRODUCT 1 (PCS)	PRODUCT 2 (PCS)	VOLUME (PCS)
CLIENT 1	19.366986	-99.053344	24000	12000	36000
CLIENT 2	19.691144	-99.212146	18000	4200	22200
CLIENT 3	19.37213	-99.098921	4800	2400	7200
CLIENT 4	19.525414	-99.103442	2400	1800	4200
CLIENT 5	19.065549	-98.103715	3000	2160	5160
CLIENT 6	19.429033	-99.136257	1200	600	1800
CLIENT 7	19.508216	-99.158846	600	360	960
CLIENT 8	19.077665	-98.155057	2400	960	3360
CLIENT 9	19.762902	-97.250398	2400	600	3000
CLIENT 10	21.067031	-101.687242	2400	480	2880
CLIENT 11	19.36011	-99.118637	1200	240	1440
CLIENT 12	18.901396	-99.227063	1440	240	1680
CLIENT 13	20.597281	-100.381743	960	360	1320
CLIENT 14	20.14495	-98.340119	600	240	840
CLIENT 15	19.509386	-101.615386	600	120	720
CLIENT 16	20.85529	-103.4462	480	240	720
		TOTAL	66480	27000	93480

Fig. 2. Customer locations

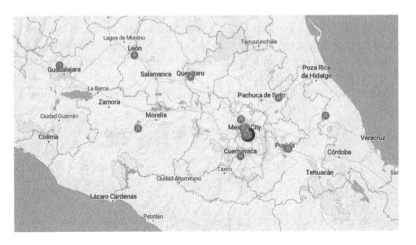

Fig. 3. Geographical customer locations

4 Simulation Models

In this section the simulation models used are presented. The process of transportation and flow of merchandise from plants to distribution centers and customers is modeled through the simulation of discrete events, see Fig. 4.

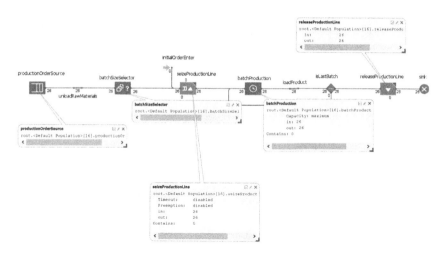

Fig. 4. Discrete-event simulation model

Agent based simulation is used to model product purchase orders by customers. This purchase order triggers production orders at the plants. The design of the supply chain is conditioned by the behavior of the purchase orders. This agent used allows considering disruptive events within it, that is, through the agent's behavior it is possible to simulate disruptive events in the supply chain. The agent based simulation is implemented in anylogic software, see [1]. Figure 5 shows the agent described above.

5 Software Used

In this work, the simulation models are implemented in a platform called AnyLogistix, which solves a variety of classic supply chain problems. The solution of these problems through simulation-optimization allows making accurate decisions in the supply chain, see [6].

The results of ALX consider the location of customers, their demands, types of products, periodicity of purchase orders, operating costs of facilities, transportation costs and inventory costs among others. So the solution obtained improves service levels, costs, profits, facility utilization rates and other key performance indicators.

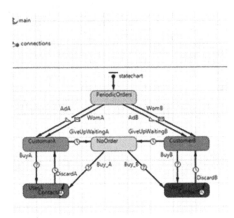

Fig. 5. Agent-based simulation model

Likewise, the proposed model allows us to analyze whether the performance indicators improve if we close, open, expand or relocate a facility. The uncertainty in the elements of the supply chain can be captured by using some ALX functions. With this uncertainty built into the analysis, the risk of supply chain operation can be assessed. The dynamic analysis allows estimating the performance of the operation as the simulation time progresses.

ALX uses analytical and simulation methods in a hybrid way to robustly model a network.

It is known that simulation techniques do not produce optimal solutions, however they allow to verify the overall performance of the system considering dynamic scenarios over time. The correlations of variables and parameters can be easily identified by running the simulation on this platform.

6   Results

Considering that ALX incorporates a georeference system, after modeling and running the simulation of the system, the results obtained show the following, see Fig. 6.

The results of the hypothetical case study show distribution centers located in different geographical areas, for example a simulation results in the location of a new distribution center at the coordinates at latitude 19.38 and longitude −99.06 coordinates.

Figure 7 shows the results for the three scenarios tested.

Figure 8 shows the distributors, the located distribution center and the supplier. The structure of supply chain is showed in Fig. 9.

SCENARIO	DESCRIPTION	X	Y
1A	Optimal location GFA	19.37	-99.05
2A	Optimal location with + 30% demand	19.38	-99.06
3A	Optimal location with + 100% demand	19.49351	-99.11

Fig. 6. Scenario results (Distribution center locations)

SCENARIO	DESCRIPTION	AVERAGE DISTANCE (km)	MINIMUM DISTANCE (km)	MAXIMUM DISTANCE (km)	DC NOT USED
1A	Optimal location GFA	100.77	4.52	477.17	DC 2
2A	+ 30% demand	109.28	4.44	477.17	DC 2
3A	+ 100% demand	237.29	2.9	2283.62	-

Fig. 7. Scenario results (distances)

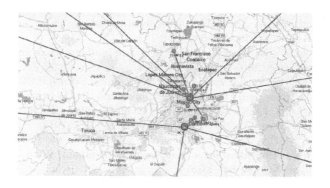

Fig. 8. Geo-referenced solution

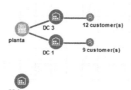

Fig. 9. Supply chain structure

7 Conclusions

This paper presents a proposal to design a supply chain. Multi-paradigm simulation is used to model the elements that make up the supply chain. Discrete event simulation is used to model the flow and transport of merchandise throughout the network as well as the operation of the distribution centers. Customer behavior is modeled through agent-based simulation and is incorporated into the global model through the AnyLogistix simulation platform. The results show that it is possible to use multiparadigm simulation to design a supply chain. As future work, the modeling of inventory policies of the distribution centers with agents that interact with the production plants can be considered.

References

1. Anylogic: Anylogic cloud (2020). https://www.anylogic.com/features/cloud/
2. Dabbene, F., Gay, P., Sacco, N.: Optimisation of fresh-food supply chains in uncertain environments, part ii: a case study. Biosys. Eng. **99**(3), 360–371 (2008)
3. Ozsen, L., Coullard, C.R., Daskin, M.S.: Capacitated warehouse location model with risk pooling. Naval Res. Logist. (NRL) **55**(4), 295–312 (2008)
4. Savadkoohi, E., Mousazadeh, M., Torabi, S.A.: A possibilistic location-inventory model for multi-period perishable pharmaceutical supply chain network design. Chem. Eng. Res. Des. **138**, 490–505 (2018)
5. Shah, N.: Pharmaceutical supply chains: key issues and strategies for optimisation. Comput. Chem. Eng. **28**(6–7), 929–941 (2004)
6. anyLogistix supply chain software: Supply chain digital twins (2020). https://www.anylogistix.com/resources/white-papers/supply-chain-digital-twins/
7. Susarla, N., Karimi, I.A.: Integrated supply chain planning for multinational pharmaceutical enterprises. Comput. Chem. Eng. **42**, 168–177 (2012)
8. Uthayakumar, R., Priyan, S.: Pharmaceutical supply chain and inventory management strategies: optimization for a pharmaceutical company and a hospital. Oper. Res. Health Care **2**(3), 52–64 (2013)

A Predictive Performance Measurement System for Decision Making in the Supply Chain

Loraine Sanchez-Jimenez$^{(\boxtimes)}$ (ID) and Tomás E. Salais-Fierro (ID)

Universidad Autónoma de Nuevo León, Pedro de Alba S/N, Ciudad Universitaria, San Nicolás de los Garza, Nuevo León, Mexico
tomas.salaisfr@uanl.edu.mx

Abstract. Increasing business competitiveness forces companies to develop strategies in search of operational excellence. The supply chain aims to increase its efficiency by reducing costs without neglecting quality and service levels. The implementation of predictive performance evaluation systems as a management practice has increased in recent years because in addition to measuring the efficiency and effectiveness of processes under certain scenarios, it includes artificial intelligence techniques that anticipate future events and allow taking advantage of behavioral patterns of historical data and current information to identify risks and opportunities. This paper proposes a fuzzy logic-based performance measurement system to help predict purchasing behavior through the impact of attributes of the SCOR supply chain operations reference model. The SCOR level 1 indicators are used as a standard for benchmarking against other supply chains. The proposed model is applied through an illustrative case and, according to the results obtained, it facilitates performance prediction and allows scenario analysis. In addition, it is adaptive to any industry and cyclical in search of the desired result, therefore, it helps decision makers to anticipate situations under uncertainty parameters and conditions by determining through simulations the performance attributes with the greatest impact on purchasing and facilitating decision making.

Keywords: Supply chain · Predictive performance measurement · Models · Fuzzy logic techniques · Logistics KPIs

1 Introduction

The most important challenge of a supply chain has is to be able to fulfill a perfect delivery in time and form adding value to the consumer. The complexity of supply chain management has been increasing over the years as many companies compete in the marketplace trying to meet customer requirements. The supply chain considers the integration of repetitive functional activities along the network that include business processes, people, technology and infrastructure for

© ICST Institute for Computer Sciences, Social Informatics and Telecommunications Engineering 2021
Published by Springer Nature Switzerland AG 2021. All Rights Reserved
J. A. Marmolejo-Saucedo et al. (Eds.): COMPSE 2021, LNICST 393, pp. 225–244, 2021.
https://doi.org/10.1007/978-3-030-87495-7_15

the transformation of raw materials into finished products and services [1]. The planning, execution and inspection of the management of goods, services and information from point of origin to point of consumption is handled by logistics [2].

The complexity of supply chain management has increased due to business competitiveness, its administration has focused on maintaining an efficient organization of activities by seeking ways to eliminate challenges through innovative strategies included in performance measurement systems. Good management practices provide competitive advantages aimed at increasing service levels, reducing inventory and improving resource utilization [3,4].

Performance measurement systems contribute to the achievement of business objectives [4]. Its structure is based on the inclusion of key indicators and metrics that evaluate the efficiency and effectiveness of the supply chain processes [5]. There are different steps to develop a performance system: identification of achievements, recording of service level, optimization of processes, objective decision making, monitoring progress and identification of areas of opportunity, control and measurement of information, evaluation and elaboration of improvement plans [6]. However, it present deficiencies in their structure when there is no connection between the strategic objectives and the metrics used, they do not do a good job when there is a biased centralization in finance or when they include conflicting measures [7], the excess of metrics and the lack of manuals for their development hinder the measurement process [8], the use of benchmarking unambiguously by comparing their performance with leading companies or companies that are not logistically similar [9]. In addition, the design, development and implementation of the performance measurement system is not a one-time practice, but must be continuously inspected and monitored to adapt to the variability of the competitive environment [10,11].

Traditional measurement systems are based on historical, independent and static information, and are less efficient in results [12]; it perform corrective actions, however, they are not ideal for measuring the variability of supply chain processes. Consequently, many researches propose the implementation of predictive performance systems that foresee future problems or needs by anticipating performance [13]. Therefore, it is essential for a supply chain to have a system that is adaptable to its needs and customized to its line of business. Performance measurement is defined as the process of quantitative and/or qualitative evaluation of the effectiveness and efficiency of an activity or business process [14].

In recent years authors have developed several supply chain performance measurement frameworks for different problems or business models [15]; based on several criteria [6]: Balanced Scorecard (BSC); components of performance measures (resources, products and flexibility); location of measures in supply chain links (plan, source, manufacture and deliver); decision levels (strategic, tactical and operational); nature of measures (financial and non-financial); basis of measures (quantitative and non-quantitative) and traditional or modern measures (function-based or value-based).

Measurements aimed at assessing cost, agility, responsiveness, flexibility, sustainability, customer and internal processes are the most popular in research [5].

The purpose of this research is to propose a predictive model to measure supply chain performance through a hybrid approach. This paper is structured in five sections: in Sect. 2, a literature review is presented for the identification of suitable tools to perform feedback to the measurement systems used by companies. Section 3 explains the proposed model, Sect. 4 presents the results obtained through the application of the illustrative case and finally Sect. 5 presents the conclusions of the study.

This article makes three contributions to the literature; first, it determines the metrics of levels 1, 2 and 3 of the SCOR model that can be implemented in the purchasing area of the supply chain. Secondly, through a benchmarking between the indicators commonly used by companies and their association with SCOR metrics, the structure of the measurement systems is evaluated, i.e., it can be determined whether the measurements performed project good results. Finally, it provides a cyclic and adaptive system for any supply chain based on a hybrid model composed of SCOR metrics and attributes, a fuzzy analytical hierarchy process for the analysis of criteria priorities and a fuzzy inference system that performs the predictive evaluation in search of identifying the performance attributes with the greatest impact in the area of study, contributing to the improvement of decision making and the formulation of action plans.

2 Literature Review

This section reviews the literature on tools used for performance measurement and provides a current analysis of the applications.

2.1 Tools to Evaluate Performance

Supply chain metrics drive performance. Erroneous assessments directly affect the key operations of any company and result in lost revenue, which in turn leads to lower long-term growth. Therefore, it is vital to use tools to measure supply chain performance. Measurement systems, frameworks, models, and techniques can be found in the literature [17,18].

The researchers [17] have followed a systematic literature review procedure on this topic, identifying the main trends in the field of supply chain performance measurement and classifying the information into approaches and techniques, also, they include the tools with the highest usage according to the search criteria contemplated: Delphi, techniques that deal with uncertainty, DEA, AHP, simulation and ANP. An update of the previous study modifies these results and includes the use of BSC, SCOR, AHP, simulation and DEA models [5]. However, a more recent article mentions AHP, DEA and fuzzy logic as the most commonly used [16].

2.2 Current Analysis of the Use of Tools

Taking into account the diagnosis presented in Sect. 2.1, a new information search is carried out. The literature review focuses on the tools used to measure some aspect or strategy of the supply chain in order to conform the hybrid model. The analysis includes 23 articles classified by author, techniques, models and artificial intelligence techniques listed in Table 1. Numbers 1 to 12 correspond to: 1: AHP, 2: ANP, 3: DEA, 4: DELPHI, 5: DEMATEL, 6: Simulation, 7: SEM, 8: BSC, 9: SCOR, 10: FUZZY, 11: Neural networks and, 12: ANFIS.

Table 1. Literature review

N	Autor	Techniques							Models		AI		
		1	2	3	4	5	6	7	8	9	10	11	12
1	Lima-Junior and Carpinetti (2020)								x				x
2	Jollembeck Lopes and I. Pires (2020)		x							x			
3	Jiang et al. (2020)	x								x			
4	Lima-Junior and Carpinetti (2019)								x			x	
5	Akkawuttiwanich and Yenradee (2018)								x	x			
6	Bukhori et al. (2015)	x								x			
7	Sellitto et al. (2015)	x								x			
8	Tavana et al. (2016)			x									
9	Wibowo and Sholeh (2016)	x									x		
10	Chand et al. (2020)				x	x							
11	Govindan et al. (2017)	x									x		
12	Rasolofo-Distler and Distler (2018)								x				
13	Thanki and Thakkar (2018)			x		x				x	x		
14	Ramezankhani et al. (2018)			x		x							
15	Haghighi et al. (2016)			x							x		
16	Tajbakhsh and Hassini (2015)			x									
17	Yu et al. (2016)			x									
18	Zanon et al. (2020)									x	x		
19	Dissanayake and Cross (2018)	x	x					x			x		
20	Tavana et al. (2016)	x											x
21	Miranda et al. (2019)						x						
22	Brandenburg (2017)	x					x						
23	Singh et al. (2018)	x								x	x		
Total		**9**	**2**	**6**	**1**	**3**	**2**	**1**	**4**	**8**	**7**	**1**	**2**

The studies were conducted in manufacturing, environmental, agricultural, construction, service and transportation companies, and the strategies implemented focused mainly on measuring sustainability in the supply chain, customer perceived value and, in other cases, supplier selection and evaluation.

Figure 1 presents the summary of the review. It can be seen that AHP, SCOR and Fuzzy Logic represent the highest utilization in supply chain measurements. However, a comparative analysis of the application of the tools in each of the categories is performed.

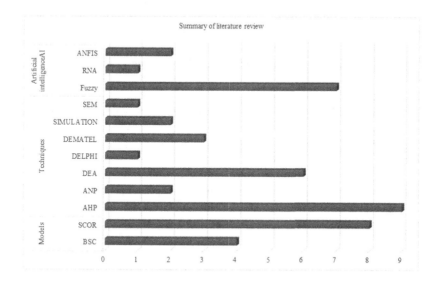

Fig. 1. Summary of literature review

The Supply Chain Operations Reference Model has a proven track record of case studies and literature research in a variety of industries. This model easily adapts to changing user requirements, effectively includes optimal metrics for assessing performance, and its criteria are compatible in a variety of supply chain contexts. As a standard model, it enables effective evaluation of supply chain performance [19]. The balanced scorecard has a history of use mainly in the financial area, however, this model has limitations because it includes fewer measures and it is complicated to measure the integrated supply chain using this approach [20]. According to this information, the model that meets the desired criteria of this study is the SCOR model.

In terms of techniques, the most widely used is the analytical hierarchical process - AHP due to its simplicity, ease of use and great flexibility. AHP consists of three main operations: hierarchy construction, priority analysis and consistency checking. It is one of the most widely used multi-criteria decision making tools and is used in selection, evaluation, cost-benefit analysis, allocations, planning and development, prioritization and ranking [21]. Data Envelopment Analysis - DEA is applied to identify sources of inefficiency, classify decision making units (DMU), evaluate management, assess the effectiveness of programs or policies, create a quantitative basis for reallocating resources, etc. [22].

On the other hand, the combination of one or more techniques is called hybrid approaches. Techniques compatible with the SCOR model are AHP, simulation and Topsis [23]. Therefore, the aggregation of AHP to the model can be considered. However, faced with the need for correct and automated decision making, the implementation of statistical or artificial intelligence (AI) techniques has increased in case investigations and illustrative tests, being employed to estimate supply chain performance based on multiple measures, to predict or check results. Adopting or combining these techniques adds new intelligent capabilities to measurement. Fuzzy logic is an approach that deals with imprecise data and knowledge, so it is ideal when historical data is not available or when decisions must be made under circumstances of uncertainty, in such cases Fuzzy AHP can be used.

The advantages of using artificial intelligence techniques transcend in the adoption of guiding metrics and related to different factors of supply chain management [24]; the ability to work with qualitative data and decision making under uncertainty [25]; adaptation to the environment [7]; and the compatibility of metrics for benchmarking [24].

To finalize the inclusion of techniques in the model, we add the application of fuzzy set theory to deal with uncertainty in the evaluation process [26]. In this regard, fuzzy inference system (FIS) has been mainly used in supply chain management problem to overcome the interior imprecision in criteria evaluation [27].

In conclusion, the hybrid model is made up of the attributes and metrics SCOR, FAHP and the fuzzy inference system with which it is intended to evaluate and provide feedback to the current measurement systems used in companies.

3   Proposed Methodology

The methodology to carry out the model is a modification of the model [28], consisting of three elements: literature review, model development and application. The modifications made are established in the configuration of the supply chain in the purchasing area based on assumptions about the SCOR performance attributes focused on the same area and the inclusion of a fuzzy AHP as a consensus technique to increase the robustness of the FIS rule design. Figure 2 illustrates the main elements of the method:

The first step is a literature review of four main theoretical concepts: performance measurement of the object of study, in this case, the purchasing area, information on the SCOR model focused on procurement attributes and indicators, the FAHP technique as a method of priority analysis and, finally, the fuzzy inference system and its applicability for supply chain performance measurement.

Secondly, the predictive performance measurement system model is developed based on the inclusion of the FAHP results as input data for the mathematical formulation of the FIS in the cause and effect relationship of the metrics.

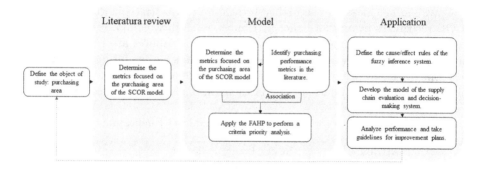

Fig. 2. Methodology

Finally, the application of the model is executed in order to demonstrate its applicability, for this, performance indicator indices and the collaboration of experts are needed to associate the SCOR model metrics with those found in the literature, subsequently measuring performance and analyzing results.

For data collection, two inputs are required in the model: current performance of the SCOR indicators focused on sourcing (information collected from literature from financial databases and articles and reports) and the second input comes from expert knowledge, which substantiates the particularities and specifics of the procurement process environment; data calculated by means of experience and linguistic scores. These data are used to form the FIS rule base.

The outputs are twofold: the current performance of the purchasing area and guidelines for improvement plans. The proposed model is cyclical in order to continuously measure different categories of the supply chain.

3.1   Theoretical Concepts

Purchasing: this area enables the company to acquire the inputs it requires with the necessary quality, in the right quantity, at the right time and at the right price. Nowadays, managers have emphasized the performance evaluation of this link; they measure and evaluate its contribution and the result is usually positive due to its ability to maximize value and minimize waste by acting proactively; improving efficiency and effectiveness in the chain [29].

The proposed methodology seeks to examine operational activities (quantitative data) and tactical and strategic activities (qualitative and less tangible data). Measurement leads to recognition of function; it establishes objectives and ground rules from which policies can be developed. In addition, benchmarking aims to discover best practices, customize them and implement them.

SCOR model: the supply chain operations reference model was introduced as a standard format that links processes, people, performance, best practices and a roadmap for supply chain excellence to meet customer demand. The performance section focuses on understanding supply chain results and constitutes two types of components: attributes; which group metrics and express specific strategies to reach a goal and, metrics; which are standard to quantify the performance of a process, i.e. measure the ability to achieve those strategic directions [19]. SCOR recognizes five performance attributes: reliability, agility, responsiveness, cost and asset management. Associated with the attributes are Level 1 strategic metrics that calculate whether an organization is successful in achieving its positioning. According to the literature review, the attributes and metrics that include source-related issues as part of their rationale are presented in Table 2.

Table 2. Performance attributes and level 1 indicators

Attribute	SCOR level 1 indicator
Realibility	Perfect order fulfilment
Agility	Upside supply chain adaptability
Asset management	Cash-to-cash cycle time
	Return on working capital
Costs	Total supply chain management costs
Responsiveness	Order fulfillment cycle time

FUZZY AHP: In seeking to understand the fuzzy nature of human reasoning, an extended version of AHP combined with fuzzy sets is proposed. This technique, known as fuzzy AHP, evaluates and classifies alternatives and has the advantage of allowing the use of appropriate linguistic values to cope with the imprecision and subjectivity of risk when making decisions [30]. The FAHP methodology is composed of several steps presented below:

– Representation for pairwise comparison: fuzzy numbers are used to model the vagueness of judgments by indicating the relative importance that one aspect has over another by means of linguistic terms and thus construct comparative matrices. Triangular fuzzy numbers (TFN's) are represented as a triplet (l,m,u) where l and u are the lower and upper values, respectively, and m is the mean value. Table 3 includes this information.

Table 3. Fuzzy AHP Saaty's scale [31]

Classic Saaty's scale	Linguistic terms	Fuzzy scale
1	Equally important	(1, 1, 1)
3	Weakly important	(2, 3, 4)
5	Fairly important	(4, 5, 6)
7	Strongly importnat	(6, 7, 8)
9	Absolutely important	(9, 9, 9)
2	Values designed for evaluation of so called interphase	(1, 2, 3)
4		(3, 4, 5)
6		(5, 6, 7)
8		(7, 8, 9)

- Synthesize the judgments: if there is more than one decision maker, it is necessary to group their preferences using the geometric mean and obtain a final result.

$$\tilde{A}_{ij} = (l_{ij}, m_{ij}, u_{ij}) = \left(\prod_{t=1}^{q} \tilde{A}_{ij}^{(t)}\right)^{\frac{1}{q}} = (\tilde{a}_{ij}^{(1)} \otimes \tilde{a}_{ij}^{(2)} \otimes \cdots \otimes \tilde{a}_{ij}^{(q)})^{\frac{1}{q}} \quad (1)$$

$$= \left(\left(\prod_{t=1}^{q} l_{ij}^{(t)}\right)^{\frac{1}{q}}, \left(\prod_{t=1}^{q} m_{ij}^{(t)}\right)^{\frac{1}{q}}, \left(\prod_{t=1}^{q} u_{ij}^{(t)}\right)^{\frac{1}{q}}\right)$$

- Calculate fuzzy weights: in this step multiple fuzzy sets of the matrix are aggregated into one by means of Eq. (2), the value of the "mean" by means of the geometric operation is then normalized to generate the fuzzy weight of a criterion, by means of Eq. (3).

$$\tilde{r}_i = [\tilde{a}_{ij} \otimes ... \tilde{a}_{in}]^{1/n} \quad (2)$$

$$\tilde{W}_i = \tilde{r}_i \otimes (\tilde{r}_1 \oplus \tilde{r}_2 \cdots \oplus \tilde{r}_n)^{-1} \quad (3)$$

- Defuzzification of fuzzy weights: converts the fuzzy results into crisp values that are more intuitive and easier for final comparison by means of the center of area (Eq. 4), then Eq. (5) is used to normalize the weights:

$$M_i = \left(l_i^W + 2m_i^W + u_i^W\right)/4, \ i = 1, 2..., n. \quad (4)$$

$$N_i = \frac{M_i}{\sum_{i=1}^{n} M_i} \quad (5)$$

- Consistency check: this step ensures that there are few contradictions between the pairwise comparison of the matrix, it is performed by means of the following equations:

$$CI = \frac{\lambda Max - n}{n - 1} \quad (6)$$

$$CR = \frac{CI}{RI} \quad (7)$$

Fuzzy inference system - FIS: is a systematic reasoning process that exposes input/output mappings using fuzzy logic to produce numerical values from linguistic values associated with membership functions [32]. It has been widely implemented in supply chain context on issues of supplier selection, supplier performance evaluation, risk, sustainability, green supply chain management, among others [33]. It has five main elements:

- A rule base composed of "IF-THEN" scenarios.
- A database of membership functions of the fuzzy sets used in the fuzzy rules.
- Decision making is an inference operation on the rules.
- A fuzzification for the transformation of crisp inputs based on linguistic values.
- A defuzzification, an operation that converts the output of the fuzzy logic into a crisp output.

3.2   Model

Figure 3 shows the proposed model that seeks to understand the impact of supply chain performance dimensions. It establishes a cyclical structure composed of three steps: determining indicators focused on the area of study, categorizing performance attributes and applying the fuzzy inference system and, finally, modeling simulation scenarios.

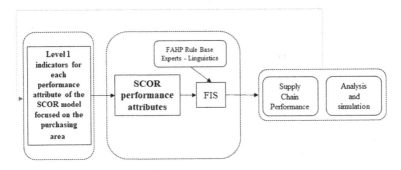

Fig. 3. Proposed model [28]

The model is configured according to the inputs, i.e., depending on the category or strategy of the supply chain to be evaluated, the applicable SCOR indicators and, therefore, the attributes are identified. The number of indicators per attribute determines the number of FIS to be performed.

4   Results

4.1   Association of Indicators

The application of the model is performed in a hypothetical case. The indicators of the purchasing area are searched in the literature and by means of the frequency in the articles contemplated 12 related in Fig. 4 are included. In the case of performing this procedure in a company, the current indicators are used.

To achieve a successful association of indicators, it is recommended to review the metrics of levels 1, 2 and 3 of the SCOR model and the description of the indicators found in the literature. After grouping these two sources, the information is simplified in such a way that it is possible to have one indicator per attribute, taking only the most relevant indicators from the literature that measure aspects of cost, inventory, delivery and quality.

Table 4 shows the final association of indicators and the conversion of figures, the current performance indexes and reference figures (taken as objective figures) are obtained from reports on the evolution of the logistics performance of supply

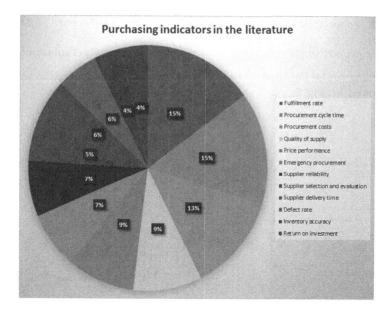

Fig. 4. Purchasing indicators in the literature

chains. In the case of applying this model in a company, these figures can be taken from the enterprise resource planning system or from the indexes of the measurement system used by the company.

Table 4. Final association of indicators and conversion of figures

SCOR level 1 indicator	Literature Indicator	Unit	Current number	Reference Figure	Proportional relationship	Converted figure (range 0–10)
Perfect order fulfillment	Compliance rate	Percentage	88	96	Direct	9
Upside supply chain adaptability	Emergency procurement	Percentage	5	3	Inverse	6
Cash-to-Cash cycle time	Return on investment	Time	6	4	Inverse	7
Return on working capital	Inventory accuracy	Percentage	80	97	Direct	8
Total supply chain managment costs	Procurement costs	Percentage	50	40	Inverse	8
Order fulfilment cycle time	Procurement cycle time	Time	6.5	4	Inverse	6

The figures are converted into a uniform range from zero to ten in order to make future internal and external benchmarking feasible. The calculation of the converted figures is carried out using the proportional relationship of the indicator with respect to performance, i.e. in the case of a direct ratio the higher the value the better the performance [28], e.g. in perfect order fulfillment and return on working capital. On the other hand, an inverse ratio refers to high figures that affect or worsen performance, as in the case of order fulfillment cycle time and the others. The following equations are used to find the values:

$$Direct\ proportional\ relationship = actual\ number/reference\ figure \qquad (8)$$

$$Inverse\ proportional\ relationship = reference\ figure/actual\ number \qquad (9)$$

According to the final association, the model to be implemented in this study is represented by Fig. 5.

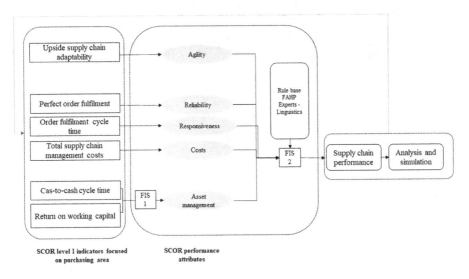

Fig. 5. Configured model

4.2   FAHP Application

In the previous section, the possible indicators used in the companies in the purchasing process were identified and associated with those of SCOR qualitatively and quantitatively. The FAHP technique is intended to determine the degree of importance of each performance attribute with respect to the area of study. These two data sources will feed the FIS rule base.

Judgments were collected by applying a survey to eleven experts in the area: people with knowledge and work experience in the field. Table 5 includes the grouping of these preferences. The acronyms correspond to RL: reliability, AG: agility, RS: responsiveness, CO: cost and AM: asset management.

The consistency ratio of this matrix is 0.016, a value suitable for the methodology. This means that there are few contradictions between the different managers considered.

Table 5. Comparison matrix for criteria

Attribute	RL			AG			RS			CO			AM		
RL	1.00	1.00	1.00	1.69	2.06	2.44	1.53	1.78	2.02	0.53	0.68	0.88	1.27	1.53	1.85
AG	0.41	0.49	0.59	1.00	1.00	1.00	0.51	0.58	0.69	0.24	0.29	0.36	0.66	0.78	0.94
RS	0.49	0.56	0.65	1.46	1.71	1.97	1.00	1.00	1.00	0.22	0.27	0.35	0.90	1.03	1.18
CO	1.13	1.48	1.90	2.77	3.43	4.13	2.84	3.70	4.52	1.00	1.00	1.00	2.73	3.22	3.74
AM	0.54	0.66	0.79	1.07	1.28	1.51	0.85	0.97	1.11	0.27	0.31	0.37	1.00	1.00	1.00

Table 6 lists the geometric means of the fuzzy comparison values of all attributes, the fuzzy weights, the total and inverse values, as well as the normalized relative weights.

Table 6. FAHP results

Attribute	ri			Wi			Mi	Ni
RL	1.116	1.305	1.518	0.169	0.230	0.312	0.235	0.230
AG	0.506	0.578	0.672	0.077	0.102	0.138	0.105	0.102
RS	0.679	0.769	0.882	0.103	0.135	0.181	0.139	0.136
CO	1.894	2.271	2.657	0.287	0.400	0.547	0.408	0.399
AM	0.666	0.759	0.865	0.101	0.134	0.178	0.137	0.133
Total	**4.861**	**5.682**	**6.593**				1.02	
Reverse (Power of -1)	0.206	0.176	0.152					
Increase order	0.152	0.176	0.206					

With the results obtained, it can be observed that the cost attribute with a relative weight of approximately 40% has the greatest relevance according to the experts' judgment in the area of supply chain purchasing, followed by reliability with 23%, while responsiveness and asset management obtain 14% and 13%, respectively. Finally, according to the results obtained, the attribute that has the least impact on the area of study is agility with 10%.

4.3 FIS Application

Two FIS are established in the model:

- FIS 1 calculates asset management from its concerning indicators. The rule base and membership functions of this first FIS are parameterized according to the experts' perception of the supply chain and the process performed by the fuzzy AHP;
- FIS 2 calculates the value of sourcing on five inputs: asset management; the consequent of FIS 1. Superior supply chain adaptability, perfect order fulfillment, order execution cycle time and total cost of supply chain management,

the level 1 indicators of agility, reliability, responsiveness and cost, respectively. It is significant to note that, in the second FIS, the rule base should be parameterized considering the purchasing value perspective.

For the two FIS defined, linguistic qualification variables are applied (Table 7).

Table 7. Linguistic terms to evaluate the antecedents and consequent [28]

Linguistic terms	TFN'S	Linguistic terms	TFN'S
Under	(0, 0, 5)	Very low	(0, 0, 2.5)
Medium	(0, 5, 10)	Low	(0, 2.5, 5)
High	(5, 10, 10)	Medium	(2.5, 5, 7.5)
		High	(5, 7.5, 10)
		Very high	(7.5, 10, 10)

Fuzzy "IF-THEN" rules are generated as a function of the antecedent linguistic variables and the number of entries. An FIS has an equal rule base ax^n, where x is the number of antecedent linguistic variables and n is the number of inputs to an FIS. The number of rules increases significantly as the number of entries increases. Therefore, 9 rules for the first FIS and 243 for the second FIS should be included in the model.

Using the procedure performed by [34], the rules are constructed based on the weights of the criteria (results of the FAHP). The proportion of the linguistic terms is determined in an interval of [0, 1] of both antecedents and consequent and the output of the rule is tilted according to the weight defined for the five linguistic terms of the consequent.

Table 8 presents the fuzzy rules for FIS 1. The same procedure is performed for the FIS 2 rules taking into account all scenarios and combinations.

Table 8. Inference rules for FIS 1

IF			THEN
Cash-to-cash time	OP	Return on working capital	Asset management
Low	AND	Low	Very low
Low	AND	Medium	Very low
Low	AND	High	Low
Medium	AND	Low	Low
Medium	AND	Medium	Medium
Medium	AND	High	High
High	AND	Low	High
High	AND	Medium	Very high
High	AND	High	Very high

The fuzzy model is based on Mamdani's algorithm and runs in the Fuzzy Logic Toolbox of the MATLAB software that develops fuzzy logic programs. Figure 6 shows the design of FIS 1 with its two input variables and the output variable.

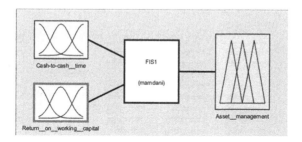

Fig. 6. FIS1 design

Figure 7 presents the rule viewer: a roadmap of the whole fuzzy inference process. The first two columns incorporate the antecedents (yellow graphs) and the third the consequent of each rule (blue graphs). Each rule is a row of graphs, and each column is a variable. The rule numbers are shown to the left of each row. The resulting graphs in the third column correspond to the aggregated weighted decision for the given inference system. This decision will depend on the input values. Finally, the result obtained in this first FIS is 6.67, a representative value of asset management from its corresponding indicators that translates to have a "medium" behavior according to the scale used. The value is determined according to the aggregation of active or executed rules (5, 6, 8 and 9, graphs with blue filling).

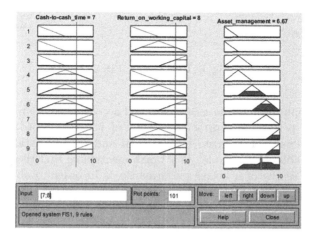

Fig. 7. Rule viewer: FIS 1 (Color figure online)

FIS 2 includes five input variables: reliability, agility, responsiveness, cost and asset management. Due to the high number of rules, Fig. 8 summarizes the output of the fuzzy system showing only the active rules, a total of 32 rules.

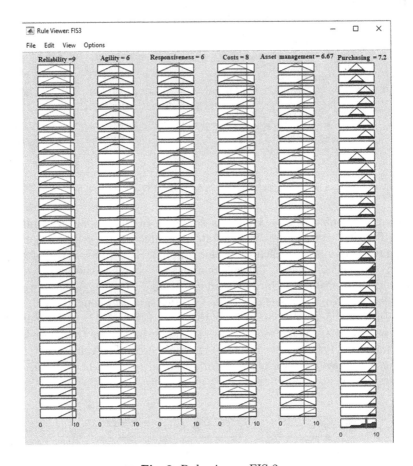

Fig. 8. Rule viewer: FIS 2

After the application of the second FIS and according to the result obtained, the purchasing performance presents a value of 7.2 determined as "medium" according to the scenarios taken into account and the evaluations entered in each of the variables of the model. It is worth mentioning that these indexes can be modified in search of a better performance or in order to obtain a desired value.

4.4   Simulation Scenarios

Following the output of FIS 2, ten comparison surfaces are generated between the attributes of the SCOR model. The plots show the three-dimensional relationship between various input and output variables. The variation of the output versus the input variables depends on the fuzzy inference rules developed. In this case, the plot of the purchasing performance as a function of the attributes is shown. This analysis helps to identify the shortest path to maximize the shopping value index. In addition, the FIS output surface provides researchers and experts with the opportunity to examine the effect of criteria on performance.

Due to the quantity, Fig. 9 presents only four cost comparison surfaces versus the other attributes because it obtained the highest contribution to purchases according to the scenario analysis.

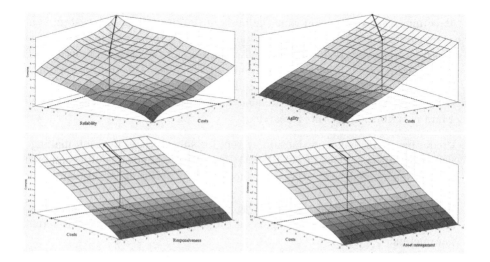

Fig. 9. Response surfaces

The behavior of very random fluctuations in the surface represents weakness and at the same time indicates an erroneous development of the generated fuzzy rules. In order to represent the sustainability and strength of the rules, the surfaces should show an approximate ascending and descending pattern. Therefore, according to the obtained behavior of few surface disturbances it can be deduced that the development of the rules was good.

In conclusion, through the analysis of all the surfaces, it is possible to deduce that the improvement mainly of costs should be essential in view of the fact that it has the greatest impact on the study area under the scenarios and parameters contemplated.

5   Conclusions

The findings reinforce the proposition that the adoption of a hybrid predictive model based on the metrics and attributes of the SCOR model with FAHP for prioritization of criteria and assignment of weights and, FIS for evaluation appears to be a viable technique to assist managers in the decision making process of supply chain performance management.

SCOR Level 1 indicators are applied as a means to evaluate the purchasing area by allowing benchmarking with other supply chains and to facilitate communication with stakeholders. The system provides the possibility of anticipation and prioritization. In addition, the model evaluates the number of indicators used in the companies and their purpose with corrective effects, also, it can take into account the variability of the processes, so it is a cyclical model in which simulations can be performed constantly varying the input data and the target goals.

It is important to mention that the basis of the fuzzy inference system is in the construction of the rules, the definition of linguistic terms and fuzzy numbers is ideal to accompany the knowledge and experience of the decision makers with a mathematical foundation through consensus techniques. The application of the FAHP for this part was successful, since it provided solidity and robustness to the rules, which was reflected in the behavior of the response surfaces.

Main contributions of this research:

- Predictive performance evaluation system for supply chain decision making.
- Hybrid model consisting of SCOR, FAHP and FIS that successfully combined and complemented each other and showed good performance measurement behavior.
- The opportunity to use the model to perform measurements in a cyclical and adaptable way for any category of the supply chain and under different parameters.
- The possibility of a corrective benchmarking for the structure (indicators) of the measurement system used by the company applying it.

References

1. Ballou, R.H.: Business Logistics Management, 4th edn. Prentice Hall, USA (1998)
2. Kozlenkova, I.V., Hult, G.T.M., Lund, D.J., Mena, J.A., Kekec, P.: The role of marketing channels in supply chain management. J. Retail. **91**(4), 586–609 (2015)
3. Qi, Y., Huo, B., Wang, Z., Yeung, H.Y.J.: The impact of operations and supply chain strategies on integration and performance. Int. J. Prod. Econ. **185**, 162–174 (2017)
4. Jayaram, J., Dixit, M., Motwani, J.: Supply chain management capability of small and medium sized family businesses in India: a multiple case study approach. Int. J. Prod. Econ. **147**, 472–485 (2014)
5. Ka, J.M.R., Ab, N.R., Lb, K.: A review on supply chain performance measurement systems. Proc. Manuf. **30**, 40–47 (2019)
6. Gunasekaran, A., Kobu, B.: Performance measures and metrics in logistics and supply chain management: a review of recent literature (1995–2004) for research and applications. Int. J. Prod. Res. **45**(12), 2819–2840 (2007)
7. Brewer, P.C., Speh, T.W.: Using the balanced scorecard to measure supply chain performance. J. Bus. Logist. **21**(1), 75–93 (2000)

8. Frazelle, E.H.: Supply Chain Strategy: The Logistics of Supply Chain Management. 1st Edition. McGraw-Hill Professional (2002)
9. Christopher, M.: Logistics and Supply Chain Management: Strategies for Reducing Cost and Improving Service, 2nd edn. Financial Times/Prentice Hall, London (1999)
10. Beamon, B.M.: Measuring SC performance. Int. J. Oper. Prod. Manage. **19**(3), 275–292 (1999)
11. Bourne, M., Mills, J., Wilcox, M., Neely, A., Platts, K.: Designing, implementing and updating performance measurement systems. Int. J. Oper. Prod. Manage. **20**(7), 754–771 (2000)
12. Lapide, L.: Predictive metrics. J. Bus. Forecast. **29**(2), 23 (2010)
13. Stefanovic, N.: Collaborative predictive business intelligence model for spare parts inventory replenishment. Comput. Sci. Inform. Syst. **12**(3), 911–930 (2015)
14. Lima-Junior, F.R., Carpinetti, L.C.R.: Quantitative models for supply chain performance evaluation: a literature review. Comput. Ind. Eng. **113**, 333–346 (2017)
15. Sundarakani, B., Razzak, H.A., Manikandan, S.: Creating a competitive advantage in the global flight catering supply chain: a case study using SCOR model. Int. J. Logist. Res. Appl. **21**(5), 481–501 (2018)
16. Lima-Junior, F.R., Carpinetti, L.C.R.: An adaptive network-based fuzzy inference system to supply chain performance evaluation based on SCOR® metrics. Comput. Ind. Eng. **139**, 106191 (2020)
17. Balfaqih, H., Nopiah, Z.M., Saibani, N., Al-Nory, M.T.: Review of supply chain performance measurement systems: 1998–2015. Comput. Ind. **82**, 135–150 (2016)
18. Beamon, B.M.: Supply chain design and analysis: models and methods. Int. J. Prod. Econ. **55**(3), 281–294 (1998)
19. APICS - Supply Chain Operations Reference Model, Version 12.0. http://www.logsuper.com/ueditor/php/upload/file/20190530/1559181653829933.pdf. Accessed 3 Mar 2017
20. Brewer, P., Speh, T.: Using the balanced scorecard to measure supply chain performance. J. Bus. Logist. **28**(1) (2000)
21. Sipahi, S., Timor, M.: The analytic hierarchy process and analytic network process: an overview of applications. Manag. Decis. **48**(5), 775–808 (2010)
22. Soheilirad, S., Govindan, K., Mardani, A., Zavadskas, E.K., Nilashi, M., Zakuan, N.: Application of data envelopment analysis models in supply chain management: a systematic review and meta-analysis. Ann. Oper. Res. **271**, 915–969 (2018)
23. Delipinar, G.E., Kocaoglu, B.: Using SCOR model to gain competitive advantage: a literature review. Proc. - Soc. Behav. Sci. **229**, 398–406 (2016)
24. Elgazzar, S., Tipi, N., Jones, G.: Key characteristics for designing a supply chain performance measurement system. Int. J. Prod. Perform. Manage. **68**(2), 296–318 (2019)
25. Najmi, A., Gholamian, M.R., Makui, A.: Supply chain performance models: a literature review on approaches, techniques, and criteria. J. Oper. Supply Chain Manag. **6**, 94–113 (2013)
26. Keshavarz Ghorabaee, M., Amiri, M., Zavadskas, E.K., Antucheviciene, J.: Supplier evaluation and selection in fuzzy environments: a review of MADM approaches. Econ. Res.-Ekonomska Istraživanja **30**(1), 1073–1118 (2017)
27. Aqlan, F., Lam, S.S.: A fuzzy-based integrated framework for supply chain risk assessment. Int. J. Prod. Econ. **161**, 54–63 (2015)
28. Zanon, L., Munhoz Arantes, R., Del Rosso Calache, L., Ribeiro Carpinetti, L.: A decision making model based on fuzzy inference to predict the impact of SCOR® indicators on customer perceived value. Int. J. Prod. Econ. **223**, 107520 (2020)

29. Baily, P., Farmer, D., Jessop, D., Jones, D.: Purchasing Principles and Management, 9th edn. Pearson, Boston (2005)
30. Adenso-Díaz, B., Alvarez, N.G., Alba, J.A.L.: A fuzzy AHP classification of container terminals. Marit. Econ. Logist. **22**, 218–238 (2020)
31. Ganesh, A.H., Shobana, A.H., Ramesh, R.: Identification of critical path for the analysis of bituminous road transport network using integrated FAHP- FTOPSIS method. Mater. Today: Proc. **37**(2), 193–206 (2021)
32. Mamdani, E., Assilian, S.: An experiment in linguistic synthesis with a fuzzy logic controller. Int. J. Man-Mach. Stud. **7**(1), 1–13 (1975)
33. Yang, M., Khan, F.I., Sadiq, R.: Prioritization of environmental issues in offshore oil and gas operations: a hybrid approach using fuzzy inference system and fuzzy analytic hierarchy process. Process Saf. Environ. Protect. **89**(1), 22–34 (2011)
34. Liu, Y., Zhang, X.: Evaluating the undergraduate course based on a fuzzy AHP-FIS model. Int. J. Mod. Educ. Comput. Sci. **12**, 55–66 (2020)

Implementation of Intelligent Automation of Production Processes in the Company Espumados del Litoral in the City of Barranquilla

Estephany Reyes, Jesus Retamozo(✉), Zaida Oliveros, Laura Sierra, Jaider Vanegas, and Carlos Jose Regalao-Noriega

Facultad de Ingenierias, Universidad SimonBolivar, Barranquilla, Atlantico, Colombia
{stephany.reyes,jesus.retamozo,zayda.oliveros,laura.sierra,
jaider.vanegas}@unisimon.edu.co, cregalao@unisimonbolivar.edu.co

Abstract. The objective of the project is to know, identify the importance and applications of the implementation of intelligent automation processes in a company, obtain a good analysis on it, to manage and integrate these digital processes in the production area of the company Espumados Del Litoral, in order to obtain a more flexible production and optimization of time.

Keywords: Automation processes · Digital processes · Production · Optimization

1 Introduction

The objective of this project is to demonstrate the importance of intelligent process automation systems and their different applications in different work areas. As we know, the main objective of process automation is to reduce costs through the integration of applications that manual processes, speeding up the execution time of tasks and eliminating the possible human errors that can be made when working manually. When optimizing a process, the following aspects must be taken into account when optimizing a process:

- i) We must know the process from end to end.
- ii) We must measure the time we are using in each task.
- iii) Analyze which aspects of the process we can eliminate or simplify.
- iv) Use software and/or applications that make our work easier. make our work easier.
- v) Integration of different platforms and software that communicate with each other.

J. A. Marmolejo-Saucedo et al. (Eds.): COMPSE 2021, LNICST 393, pp. 245–251, 2021.
https://doi.org/10.1007/978-3-030-87495-7_16

2 Development

2.1 Problem Statement

The problem posed for the development of the project aims to answer the following question: What computer-simulated solution alternatives based on and based on industrial automation tools can be automation tools can be implemented in Espumados del Litoral S.A.? In order to improve the efficiency of the improve the efficiency of production processes the industrial engineering career offers different analysis tools and seeks to propose and implement improvement plans and provide solutions to specific situations, both in the specific situations, both in the operational and administrative areas, as well as administrative. This means that every process can be improved, but it is be improved, but it is important to give priority to those with long execution times, high costs or those that show high costs or that show a competitive difference through the use of technology competitive difference through the use of advanced technology. One of the basic technological tools for process for process improvement is automation and our focus in this case is the automation and our focus in this case is the operative area of the company operational area of the company Espumados del Litoral S.A. Which, as a production plant, is looking for alternative solutions to implement improvements in the efficiency of the production processes based on industrial automation tools.

Today, the country's purchasing power has improved has improved, helping to import and create new import and creation of new products that products that make people's lives more comfortable people's lives, evolving the companies to satisfy the needs of the consumer. In the course of time, the company of Espumados del Litoral, has been recognized has been recognized and has undergone great changes. In fact, by means of capital flows and machinery necessary to manufacture flexible foams, with the passage of time, the national market has been expanding and so did its consumption by the mattress, upholstery and the mattresses, footwear, etc., resulting in a satisfied demand. resulting in a satisfied demand. In Latin Latin America, the uses and applications of flexible polyurethane foams are represented polyurethane foams are represented in a 57% for the upholstery and the upholstery and mattress sector, 10% in the automotive area, 16% in the automotive, 16% for rigid - sprayed foams and 17% for various uses, such as thermal insulation, adhesives insulation, adhesives, sealants and elastomers, giving an idea of the number of an idea of the number of applications and uses in our daily life [1]. However, there are currently several ways of manufacturing flexible polyurethane foams in small and large scale, taking into account the volume of sales, thus trying to of sales, thus trying to cover the foaming market in the city of Bariloche the foaming market in the city of Barranquilla and generate employment, since the volume of consumption is increasing in Latin America and the world, for this reason it is proposed the realization the realization and implementation of intelligent automation to obtain a good analysis on this, to manage and integrate these digital processes digital in the production area of the company Espumados del Litoral.

3 A Look at Automatic Control

3.1 Introduction to Automatic Control

Intelligent automation and control processes have been gaining momentum in recent years, thanks to the progress and development of technology. Although since the industrial revolution, process optimization and operating cost optimization and savings in operating costs, the current dynamics have driven the current dynamics have driven the generation of different mechanisms to increase productivity and competitiveness, incorporating mechanical, electronic and mechanical, electronic and computerized systems that are replacing manual labor.

In the third and last stage, the analysis of the information is performed information in order to design a report that will allow students to students to identify which are the managerial competencies and skills that should be managerial competencies and skills that should be applied in a managerial role. Automatic control has played a vital role in the advancement of engineering and science. In addition its extreme importance in spacecraft, missile guidance, robotic space vehicles, and similar systems, automatic control has robotics and the like, an important integral part of modern industrial and manufacturing processes. For example, automatic control is control is essential in the numerical control of machine tools in manufacturing industries, in the design of manufacturing industries, autopilot systems in the aerospace industry, and in the design of cars and trucks design in the automotive industry. It is also essential in industrial operations such as pressure, temperature, humidity, viscosity and flow control in the humidity, viscosity and flow in the process industries process industries.

Process control and automation are appearing in the world and have been advancing since the beginning of the industrial revolution; although the term as such has been the term, it refers to the ability of technology to carry out technology's capacity out work or daily life processes with work with a high degree of ease and effectiveness, saving and effectiveness, saving resources, physical effort and time. It is essential for the economic progress of and explore new methods in production and logistical in production, especially those based on new technologies, in order to reach the levels of competitiveness required in an increasingly globalized market. It is estimated, according to the McKinsey Global Institute, that automation levels can range from 41% to 55%, with between 41% and 55%, with the developed and emerging countries that have implemented automation methods and tools in their industries that can automation tools that can replace, according to the same study, some 1.2 billion jobs worldwide, which is undoubtedly a challenge for the undoubtedly a challenge for states, companies and educational institutions [2]. Regarding the ranking of robot implementation, for example, to industrial processes, leading the list are South Korea, Singapore and Japan lead the list; Mexico, Argentina and Brazil are the first in Latin America [3]. Understanding, therefore, the phenomena related to control and intelligent automation allow the public and private sectors to make decisions on the implementation of such processes, taking into account the social, political and social economic impacts that may be generated impacts that may be generated.

3.2 Definition of Control and Intelligent Automation

Intelligent control and automation is understood as the system that collects data, processes it and generates autonomous orders that allow the inspection, control and intervention of environments and communication with users. Throughout the history of humankind, man has sought to adapt the world to its conditions, while other species have simply adapted to it [4]. This particular characteristic of the human being has been an engine of innovation and entrepreneurship that continually modifies society's way of continuously modifies the way of life of society and even of other species. The use of animals for transportation, the invention of the wheel, writing, mathematics, agriculture, electricity, communications and the computer, among others, have been inventions that have led mankind to humanity to transmute physical energy into time to continue creating and innovating into time to continue creating and innovating; time that is in today's society as a high-value resource.

3.3 The Power of Automation in Organizations

Advances in technical developments in computer hardware and software have made it possible to introduce automation into virtually all aspects of human-machine systems [5]. This science not only replaces physical matter, but also brings about changes in the activities carried out by human beings [6] refers to the total or partial substitution of a function, previously performed by human beings, with the possibility of varying the level of application, i.e. whether the process is slightly or highly automated. To better understand the concept of automation, the Royal Academy of Exact, Physical and Natural Sciences (RA-CEFyN) of Spain starts from the definition of automation, understood as the set of methods and procedures for the replacement of the operator in physical and mental tasks and previously programmed, therefore, automation is understood as the application of automation to the control of industrial processes and has evolved to many fields of science. The Dictionary of the Royal Spanish Academy [15], derives it to the verb to automation the same that has two meanings: on the one hand, "to convert certain movements into automatic or in deliberate movements", and, on the other hand, "to apply the automatic to a process or a device". It also rescues the definition of the Oxford English Dictionary [16], when it refers that automation is the action or process of introducing automatic equipment or devices in a factory or other process or facility, or also as the fact of doing something through a system, device, etc. automatically. Furthermore, since the 1950s it was related to mechanical or electronic devices and allowed the substitution of people's work, which has remained to the present day. For Parasuraman et al. [7] automation refers to the total or partial substitution of a function, previously performed by human beings, and the level of application may vary, i.e. whether the process is slightly or highly automated. In another research Parasuraman and Riley [14] define automation as a concept that can change over time, under the conception that automation comes from a machine (usually a computer) and where the assignments of functions from human to machine will be transferred and will change over time. There are several criteria regarding the roots of automation, for Sergio Parra [8] they go back to very ancient times before Christ: In the eighth century BC, Homer, in his famous Iliad, already describes mechanical servants endowed with intelligence built by Hephaestus, the god of metallurgy.

Between 400–350 B.C., Archytas of Tarentum built an automatic bird. Between 262–190 B.C., Apollonius of Perga invented a series of water-powered musical automata Ctesibius also built musical automata, whose sound was created by the passage of air through various tubes. According to Macau [9], one of the first milestones that marked the history of automation is that "from 1960 onwards, information technology was introduced into organizations with the aim of automating repetitive administrative tasks (mainly accounting, invoicing and payroll)", transforming the organizational processes of companies from that time to the present day. The next big step, which occurred at the end of the 1970s, according to Rafael Macau [10] was the emergence of the concept of "Management Information System (MIS), an integrated information system that, based on a global design, comprises both bureaucratic work automation systems and management information systems for the different management levels" within an organization. For Gerardo Tunal [11] automation has two origins dating back to the 1980s. The first was when the statistician of the U.S. Census Bureau [18], Herman Hollerith [19], created a computer capable of classifying punched cards, duplicating and comparing them and being able to code population data to generate census statistics, and the second milestone, when in 1994 Howard H. Aiken [20], of the University of California, Berkeley, USA, created a computer that could be used to generate census statistics [12]. Aiken, from Harvard University, created the first fully automatic and electronic calculator, the Automatic Sequence Controlled Calculator (ASCC), with which it was possible to perform continuous operations previously programmed [17]. These inventions had a high value for the time due to the conditions in which they were developed and the technological advances, the first one has even been considered as a preordained one.

4 Methodology

The development of the present research was elaborated under a systemic literature review methodology. The systemic literature review provides the facility to identify, contrast, evaluate and interpret the relevant research available and on that to answer certain research questions that have been posed, which can be one or more than one [13]. The purpose of using this methodology is to identify current research with respect to intelligent process automation and to find new areas or lines of research for future research. A protocol was used that includes the following elements: Problem statement, State of the art and Objectives.

5 Conclusions and Discussions of Information Analysis

We can conclude that because automation systems most of the time are very complex and diverse. The proposed methodology provides a useful tool to carry out automation projects. But in order to successfully carry out an automation project it is necessary to obtain in the greatest detail the information of the system description, since this is the one that opens all the gaps to acquire the (existing) technology, in addition to helping to have a broad vision of what can and wants to do. The solutions found for the present investigation are framed in the themes of Cost reduction:

i)   Improvement in equipment load, decreasing resources.
ii) Reduction in the number of errors: Human or communication errors.
iii) Significant increase in execution speed: Significant time reduction.
iv) Obtaining reports: Quickly and on the spot.

References

1. Alfaro, S.C., Drews, P.: Intelligent systems for welding process automation. J. Braz. Soc. Mech. Sci. Eng. **28**(1), (2006)
2. Berruti, F., Nixon, G., Taglioni, G., Whiteman, R.: Intelligent process automation: the engine at the core of the next-generation operating model. Digital Mckinsey (2017)
3. Ortega Morocho, R.J.: Diseño y construcción de un prototipo de ascensor inteligente controlado por un PLC para el laboratorio de Automatización Industrial de procesos Mecánicos. Proyecto de grado, EPN. Quito (2013)
4. Jimenez Macías, E.: Técnicas de Automatización Avanzadas en Procesos Industriales. Ph Doctoral, Departamentos de Matemáticas y Computación y de Ingeniería Eléctrica, Universidad de la Rioja, Logroño (2004)
5. Beltran Gaxiola, M.T.: Impacto Laboral por la Automatización en los Procesos productivos en la 1 Industria Automotriz de Sonora: Caso Ford 1990–2017. M.S. Thesis, Universidad de Sonora. Hermosillo, Sonora (2020)
6. Quintana, B., Pereira, V., Vega, C.: Automatización en el hogar: Un proceso de diseño para viviendas de interés social. Revista EAN (78), 108–121 (2015)
7. Institución Universitaria Esumer: Control y Automatización Inteligente (2018). http://repositorio.esumer.edu.co/jspui/handle/esumer/1903
8. Valdiviezo-Abad, C., Bonini, T.: Automatización Inteligente en la gestión de la comunicación. Doxa Comunicación **29**, 169–196 (2019)
9. Balanzá, J., Gonzales, R., Busquet, J.: Controlador inteligente para la Automatización del control de pozos petroleros. México (2015)
10. García Moreno, E.: Automatización de procesos industriales: robótica y automática. Valencia: Editorial de la Universidad Politécnica de Valencia (2020). https://ezproxy.unisimon.edu.co:2258/es/lc/unisimon/titulos/129686
11. Ángel, N., Daladier, J., Garyn, C., José, C.: Influencia de la Ingeniería de Software en los Procesos de Automatización Industrial. Información tecnológica (2019). https://scielo.conicyt.cl/scielo.php?script=sci_arttext&pid=S071807642019000500221&lng=en&nrm=iso&tlng=en
12. Arbelaez, J., Rodriguez, C., Hincapie, D., Simanca, P., Torres, E., Upegui, A.: Intervención tecnológica para la reconversión y automatización de una máquina termo formadora por vacío de una solaestación (2019)
13. Moreno, J.: La automatización de los procesos y el trabajo humano (2016)
14. Camargo, B., Duran, B., Rosa, J.: Plataforma hardware/software abierta para aplicaciones en procesos de automatización industrial (2013)
15. Niño, L., Méndez, Fuquen, H.: Automatización de procesos en la central Chivor para monitoreo y control de variables críticas (2015)
16. Diaz, P., Diaz, G., Brunet, A.: Sistema automatizado para el control de las inversiones en las redes eléctricas (2015)
17. Adolfo, M., Deimer, P., Sánchez, G.: Un prototipo mecánico para la automatización del proceso de selección del mango tipo exportación (2012)
18. Castillo, H., Echeverry, A., Zapata, A.: Desarrollo de un Sistema automatizado y de control remoto para un reactor mono evaporador de arco pulsado (2006). file:///C:/Users/Usuario/Documents/ContentServer%20(1).pdf

19. Liorni, F.: Procedimiento general para la instrumentación del proyecto de automatización industrial en la empresa azucarera "Ifraín Alfonso" (2009)
20. Ponsa, P., Villanueva, G., Diaz, M.: Introducción del operario humano en el ciclo de automatización de procesos mediante la guía GEMMA (2007)

A Look at the Literature Review of the Impact of Industry 4.0 on the Logistics Processes of the Food Sector in Barranquilla

Carolina Rangel, Jose Otero[✉], Frency Antequera, Yuliana Bonadiez, Mary Riquett, and Carlos Jose Regalao-Noriega

Facultad de Ingenierías, Universidad Simón Bolívar, Barranquilla, Atlántico, Colombia
{carolina.rangel,jotero6,Frency.antequera,yuliana.bonadiez,
Mary.riquett}@unisimon.edu.co, cregalao@unisimonbolivar.edu.co

Abstract. Industry 4.0 or fourth industrial generation, is well known as the Internet of Things (IOT) which is a means of communication for humans that will allow us to have many intelligent systems for business that help the collection and use of data in the cloud, this will bring us many improvements for the search for solutions in manufacturing and logistics processes. That is, with the advent of this industry, technology has played an important role in the modernization of logistics processes. Digital platforms have allowed the distribution processes of goods to become faster, more efficient, reliable and economical. This Industry 4.0 is an excellent strategy to implement in the food sector of Barranquilla, since it meets the basic needs in relation to logistics, such as the high need for transparency and integrity control along the supply chain (right products, at the right time, place and right quantities and at a good price) which greatly benefits food companies since this fourth industry helps to adapt to the needs of customers, to improve the distribution of products and to be more efficient in delivery times.

Keywords: Suppliers · Supply chain · Technology · Blockchain

1 Introduction

Through the different resources and strategies that industry 4.0 offers us, we find a number of applications that have allowed us to evolve, we implement the investigation of industry 4.0 within the logistics processes in the food sector in Barranquilla, focusing our research on the optimization of these resources for the common good. Industry 4.0 has been one of the most relevant technologies for these years, that is why we seek to know and learn how beneficial these technologies can become in the aforementioned sector. In view of this, its importance lies in the fact that it can supply people in its totality and provide great information to each of the companies that would use it to solve problems faster and more efficiently. Therefore, the efficiency of 4.0 technology can be of great benefit to these food companies, as it would reduce the price of different fields that are developed as the production, delivery time and product development.

© ICST Institute for Computer Sciences, Social Informatics and Telecommunications Engineering 2021
Published by Springer Nature Switzerland AG 2021. All Rights Reserved
J. A. Marmolejo-Saucedo et al. (Eds.): COMPSE 2021, LNICST 393, pp. 252–258, 2021.
https://doi.org/10.1007/978-3-030-87495-7_17

Considering that it is an advanced technology, we have to know how would be the process for the implementation of some of its tools, as it would be the Big data; since it is the main source that is applied in this industry for the elaboration of each of the tasks that we want to implement. Through this research, we managed to know how important it is to have a great team that projects and drives our knowledge, supplying our needs and embracing a future full of technology that would allow us to be competent human beings and able to be at the height of industry 4.0; the new digital era. thus leading us to enter an industry 4.0 in an active society full of technology, a society enabled and prepared to meet their own needs through technology. The fourth industrial revolution prepares us and introduces us to a new world full of technology; in order to instill in us knowledge that allows us to create strategies to make our lives easier. From the above, the objective is set in supplying the basic needs in relation to logistics such as control and transparency in industry 4.0; such as creating intelligent systems for businesses that help the collection of food to find improvements in the database for the manufactures and distribution of goods efficiently in the industry and evaluate the implementation and efficiency of the company in the productivity processes in the food area.

2   Industry 4.0 in the Food Sector

Industry 4.0 and the food industry [1] have advantages that the fourth industry has, the technological advances that it has are incorporated by companies in developed countries. And in them, support programs have been implemented for the adoption of these new technologies. There are similar actions in developing countries. The food industry is also integrated into these trends. This has been done because through the use of these technologies, companies improve their quality, reduce processing and delivery time to customers, as well as product customization. Therefore, it is very important to take into account the implementation of these technologies because in the food industry there are many changes in different aspects: in consumption patterns, in tastes and preferences, in quality and sanitation requirements, price, among other aspects. It is therefore important for companies to be aware of all the technological advances that enable them to be flexible and respond quickly to consumer needs or preferences and to changes in consumption patterns in order to remain and grow in the market. Effects generated by the application of logistics 4.0 in the supply chain of the food industry sector in Colombia. The growth of the Colombian food production industry which is considered of weight in the economic sectors, since in recent years it provides almost 21.23% of the Manufacturing GDP and 2.83% of the total GDP that forms a duo with logistics 4.0 creating a strong sector that forecasts an important economic positioning of the nation in Latin America.

Among these tools is the Big data that is used to improve the logistics movements of the warehouse. Data that can come from various sources. The most common data sources are: Vehicle diagnostics, Traffic and weather data. Although there are also some challenges with logistics 4.0, one obstacle is the infrastructure in Colombia, this is with problems both in roads and railways, ports and airports, which has caused the country to be positioned in this area at lower levels compared to other countries in Latin America and the rest of the world. The new paradigm of Industry 4.0 and its application to the agri-food industry [2]. Here they took as a reference a company in the food sector, focusing on this industry, to analyze the new opportunities and challenges, since in order to meet the new expectations, industrial organizations need an automated process to deliver plant information to a higher corporate level in an accurate, standardized, efficient and secure way. To this end, industry relies on so-called technology enablers. Industry 4.0 has all these characteristics. So, in order to relate this technology to the food company that was used as an example, the first thing to do was to identify the problems that the company has:

1. Demand prediction Predictive maintenance Energy management: The development of new ICT-based systems and tools makes it possible to improve energy efficiency in all sectors, optimize and improve energy management, active demand management and electric mobility. Incorporation of industry 4.0 in the primary link of the dairy chain in the department of Cundinamarca [3]. (Cundinamarca, June 5, 2019) Incorporation of industry 4.0 in the primary link of the dairy chain in the department of Cundinamarca. [Online] http://repositorio.uniagustiniana.edu.co/handle/123456 789/848 The Colombian dairy subsector has grown in recent times thanks to industry 4.0, expanding as an important exporter, although it is still far from the world leaders it has been positioning itself. Constantly, the world dairy subsector is changing, any movement of the world powers has an impact on the country.

Because of this, it is essential that the subsector be more competitive in order to be able to satisfactorily face the current obstacles in a globalized world. To this end, it is believed that the sector should maintain a good relationship with the state, consolidating and strengthening its ties in order to reach agreements that ensure better sustainability while the sector lays more appropriate foundations that allow an increase in efficiency, productivity and quality. Aspiring in the future to be one of the leading countries in the world.

Determinants of the financial structure in the manufacturing industry: the food industry [4] determinants of the financial structure in the manufacturing industry: This article aims to determine the mechanisms and firm-specific variables of the financial structure of firms belonging to the food industry in Mexico during the period 2000–2009. A clustered ordinary least squares econometric analysis is developed to identify these variables, which shows that tangible assets are the main variable that these firms consider to define their financing decisions.

From Industry 4.0 to Agriculture 4.0: Current Status, Enabling Technologies and Research Challenges [5, 6]. From Industry 4.0 to Agriculture 4.0: Current Status, Enabling Technologies, and Research This article shows how the industrial revolutions have transformed agriculture, where productivity has improved and where a reform is expected to promote the fourth agricultural revolution. It also shows the production patterns, processes and the supply chain, where 5 technologies are discussed, some of them are: robotics and artificial intelligence. This article was conducted for the purpose of new research opportunities.

From industry 4.0 to society 4.0, there and back [7, 8]. From industry 4.0 to society 4.0, there and back. This article discusses the links between digital society, digital culture and Industry 4.0. More precisely it examines the change that workers are subject to, along with the organization of work, smart digital factories. In the article they wanted to highlight that the elements of Industry 4.0 are widespread in addition to the factory, in society, which are not only technological elements but also cultural. For it is a transformation that contributes to the integration of digital communication technologies (digital media) in industrial processes, reinventing products, services and production methods.

Industry 4.0 in the digital society [9]. Industry 4.0 in the digital society. In this one, they address the issue of the technologies that Industry 4.0 has and the impact of its arrival, highlighting that many of the technological advances that form the basis of the fourth industry are already used in the current factory of what is known as Industry 3.0, but when the new 4.0 model is implemented in its entirety, we will see a very large transformation in production, everything will become a fully integrated, automated and optimized production flow, and will lead the factory to greater efficiency and productivity. The traditional interrelationships between suppliers, producers and customers will undergo major changes, as will the relationships between humans and machines. Some of the Industry 4.0 technologies that in the article were shown as in a diagram and showed a connection between all, are: Autonomous robots, simulation, horizontal and vertical integration, Internet of things, Cybersecurity, Cloud computing, augmented reality, Big data.

Human food, pig farming, industry 4.0, analytics, internet of things, big data, sensors. With the technological advances as a result of industry 4.0 in the food sector has shown that in the world there is a need to produce food to meet the demand of the growing population. Animal protein is the most bioavailable food source (best assimilation) for the human body due to its contribution of essential amino acids. Estado de la Industria 4.0 en el sector alimentario andaluz [10]. The food industry is important in the economic system of Andalusia, as it stimulates its advantages and potentialities, which enhances opportunities for improvement.

Industry 4.0 is a necessity for the industry in general that seeks to redesign a smart factory with advances in the field that incorporate greater flexibility and individualization in manufacturing processes.

Industry 4.0 Internet of Things. In this article we talk about the beginnings of the industry 4.0 that were in Germany exactly in the year 2011 and well in a few words they describe it as an intelligence factory since it is achieved that all processes are interconnected through the internet of things as it is also known to this industry 4.0 and it is a process that points to what would be the next level of the industrial revolution since it will be able to drive fundamental changes that are at the height of the first, second and third revolution [13]. In this case, this fourth industry will represent an evolution of the industry, all by merging the factory with the internet, through the design and implementation of intelligent components. In short, it can be said that the main objective of Industry 4.0 is to ensure that machines remain interconnected, analyzing information and designing new business models and manufacturing systems on their own.

Industry 4.0 in logistics processes. In this article they start by defining industry 4.0, they expose it as a technology that includes digitization, interconnection and cloud computing [11]. They also highlight that, the Internet of Things promises far-reaching payoffs for companies, logistics operators, their customers and end consumers. These benefits

extend across the entire value chain, including warehousing, operations, freight forwarding, among others. The connected industry 4.0. This article emphasizes the implications
of industry 4.0 in aspects of the economy and all those results that digital transformation
can bring for industrial companies [12]. They detail the significant difference that this
industry has had in relation to the past ones, in that those three revolutions introduced
greater or lesser improvements in the productive processes along the value chain and,
nevertheless, none of them demonstrated the transforming capacity that the interconnection of machines [15], products, suppliers and millions of consumers implies; and on the
other hand, because the transformation that is taking place has as distinctive signs also
the great speed with which it is developing and the framework of integral connectivity
in which it is taking place [16].

Industry 4.0 in Latin America: A roadmap for its implementation. In this we mention
the application that this technology has in different countries, in which, Europe, USA,
and countries of the Far East as their large companies lead this implementation according
to automation standards [14]. A different case in Latin America, more specifically in
small and medium enterprises, which have problems ranging from ignorance of the
technology, rigid business structures, training of human resources, lack of standards,
which creates a great risk for them in their incorporation.

That said, the purpose for them was to establish a route that can be followed for
the implementation of Industry 4.0 and for this the following elements must be followed: Motivators, enablers and knowledge.Análisis del sector lechero y aplicaciones
tecnológicas de la industria 4.0

3 Methodology

The method of the project is framed within the research line of Operations Management
in terms of the study of the thematic axis of supply chains from the perspective of
the insertion of technologies in organizational logistics processes. From a process of
observation and direct analysis to determine the factors that influence decision-making on
the absorption of 4.0 technologies in the case of the food sector in the city of Barranquilla.
Based on the above, a three-phase research process is proposed:

i)   It begins with a general characterization of the companies studied taking as a ref-
     erence the analysis of vertical and horizontal integration systems in the framework
     of industry 4.0. This is a snapshot of the current reality of the object of study.
ii) Then, by means of the computer package and the use of the statistical tool, the
     factors and variables under study in this project are established.
iii) The factors that allow evaluating the impact of Industry 4.0 technologies and that
     have a significant impact on the logistics processes of the food sector in the city of
     Barranquilla are quantitatively established.

4 Expected Results

With the analysis and data obtained in the research in the food sector, it is intended to
obtain 3 very important elements for the benefit of the companies, which are:

i)   Optimization at the moment of distributing food quantities.
ii) The quality that is realized in the logistic process for the distribution of food products.
iii) The time saved by each one of the machines and strategies according to the indicators drawn for the sector.

5   Conclusions and Discussions of Information Analysis

Industry 4.0 or better known with the Internet of Things (IoT) presents new ways of seeing different things for the digitization and growth of this in the food sector, incorporating new technological advances in underdeveloped countries, these technologies have made companies have an improvement in product quality.

Taking with them the big data tools that help us to improve the logistic movements of the warehouses, we can mention that this technology has helped different countries such as Latin America, Far East countries, among others.

Further on the financial structures in the manufacturing industry has as a mechanism to develop econometric analysis of clustered ordinary least squares that allows us to identify these variables, which shows whether these samples are the main variables that consider determining the decisions of a company.

Continuing with this, industry 4.0 in the food and manufacturing sector has as its current state, great challenges in productivity and the supply chain, which is reformed from the 4th industrial revolution and is bringing with it great technologies that include robotics, artificial intelligence, among others; with advances in the field that incorporate greater flexibility and individualization in manufacturing processes.

In conclusion, society, digitization culture and logistics 4.0, examines the changes that can be in a company with intelligent technology, beyond touching it is worth noting that not only the technological elements are important for society, but also the culture, as this helps us to get to transform processes, which contribute to the integration of technology of industrial means, reinventing products, services and production methods.

Finally, all interconnected processes can be achieved through the internet of things, due to this can achieve a great change in the industrial revolution. If it continues in this way, it can be said that IoT promotes far-reaching rewards for companies, logistics operators, their customers and end consumers.

References

1. Trejo, A.R., Alquicira, A.M., Mondragón, I.J.G.: La industria 4.0 y la industria alimentaria (24 marzo 2020). [En línea]. Disponible en: https://www.riico.net/index.php/riico/article/view/1830
2. Iván, Q., César, B.: Revisión sistemática de literatura: efectos generados por la aplicación de la logística 4.0 en la cadena de suministros del sector industria de alimentos en Colombia (18 agosto 2020). [En línea]. Disponible en: https://repository.ucc.edu.co/handle/20.500.12494/20285
3. Manuel, G., Amalia, L., Juan, L.: El nuevo paradigma de la industria 4.0 y su aplicación a la industria agroalimentaria (2018). [En línea]. Disponible en: https://idus.us.es/handle/11441/88922

4. González Patiño, V.: Incorporación de la industria 4.0 en el eslabón primario de la cadena láctea del departamento de Cundinamarca, Cundinamarca, junio 5 de (2019). [En línea]. http://repositorio.uniagustiniana.edu.co/handle/123456789/848

5. Carmen, G.H., Bolívar, H.R.: Determinantes de la estructura financiera en la industria manufacturera: la industria de alimentos (abril 2012). [En línea]. https://www.redalyc.org/pdf/413/41324594006.pdf

6. Liu, Y., Mamá, X., Shu, L., Hancke, G.P., Abu-Mahfouz, A.M.: From Industry 4.0 to Agriculture 4.0: Current Status, Enabling Technologies, and Research Challenges (2020). [En línea]. Disponible en: https://ezproxy.unisimon.edu.co:2091/record/display.uri?eid=2-s2.0-85102352274&origin=resultslist&sort=plff&src=s&st1=&st2=&sid=5303b43081490e06c6a922a39a0d0825&sot=b&sdt=b&sl=32&s=TITLE-ABSKEY%28food+industry+4.0%29&relpos=0&citeCnt=1&searchTerm=

7. Tatiana, M.: From industry 4.0 to society 4.0, there and back (August 2018). https://ezproxy.unisimon.edu.co:2102/10.1007/s00146-017-0792-6

8. Garrell, A., Guillera, L.: La industria 4.0 en la sociedad digital (2019). [En línea]. Disponible en: https://books.google.es/books?hl=es&lr=&id=YnSIDwAAQBAJ&oi=fnd&pg=PA51&dq=La+industria+4.0+en+la+sociedad+digital.&ots=tef6qF663s&sig=HPTodtUsTw_9CI-xoJ1ALQNPPKs

9. Hincapié Pineda, S.: masterThesis: Industria 4.0 en el sector porcicola y los avances alimenticios (2020). [En línea] Disponible en: https://repository.upb.edu.co/bitstream/handle/20.500.11912/6148/Alimentación%20humana%2c%20porcicultura%2c%20industria%204.0%2c.pdf?sequence=1&isAllowed=y

10. Luque, M.: Estela Peralta - A. de las Heras - A. Córdoba Estado de la Industria 4.0 en el sector alimentario andaluz, Andalucía (2017). [En línea] Disponible en https://www.sciencedirect.com/science/article/pii/S235197891730834X

11. Verónica, T.: Industria 4.0- Internet de las cosas [En línea] (2017). Disponible en: http://investigacion.utc.edu.ec/revistasutc/index.php/utciencia/article/view/6

12. МО После́д: Industria 4.0 en procesos logísticos [En línea] (2020). Disponible en: https://rep.bntu.by/bitstream/handle/data/77122/308-311.pdf?sequence=1

13. Mario, B., Fernando, V.: La industria conectada 4.0 (2017). [En línea]. Disponible en: https://e4-0.ipn.mx/wp-content/uploads/2019/10/la-industria-conectada-4-0.pdf

14. Edgar, C., Juan, C., Julián, U.: Industria 4.0 en América Latina: Una ruta para su implantación, 01 January 2020. [En línea]. Disponible en: https://revistas.ufps.edu.co/index.php/ingenio/article/view/2386

15. Lorena, B.: Industria 4.0 Y La Gestión De La Cadena De Suministro: El Desafío De La Nueva Revolución Industrial (2018). [Enlínea]. Disponible en: http://publicaciones.usm.edu.ec/index.php/GS/article/view/103

16. Manuel, G., Amalia, L., Juan, L.: Técnicas de predicción mediante minería de datos en la industria alimentaria bajo el paradigma de Industria 4.0 (2019) [En línea]. Disponible en: https://idus.us.es/handle/11441/88838

Author Index

Acasuso, Saul Fernando Peregrina   216
Alarcón-Bernal, Zaida Estefanía   162
Andrade-Gonzalez, Rosalia   73
Antequera, Frency   252
Arredondo, José Luis Hernández   28
Arrioja-Castrejón, Edmundo   143

Bernal, Zaida Estafanía Alarcón   28
Bonadiez, Yuliana   252

Callejas, Gerardo Meza   216

de Asís López-Fuentes, Francisco   63
del Carmen Daza Guerra, Helia Rosa   196
DelaTorre-Díaz, Lorena   88
De-los-Santos Ventura, Cristina   3

Enríquez-Martínez, Valeria   12

Gao, Xinyu   45
Girault, Juan Pablo Gutierrez   216
González-Badillo, Itzel Viridiana   162

Jimenez-Angeles, Luis   129

Liu, Xinyang   109
López-Fernández, Andrée Marie   143

Marcelín-Jiménez, Ricardo   63
Marmolejo-Saucedo, José A.   12
Marmolejo-Saucedo, Jose Antonio   129, 216

Niembro-García, Isabel J.   12

Oliveros, Zaida   245
Ortega-Vallejo, Raúl Antonio   63

Ortiz-Ospino, Luis   177
Otero, Jose   252

Pan, Shuning   45
Pourroostaei Ardakani, Saeid   45, 109

Rangel, Carolina   252
Regalao-Noriega, Carlos Jose   177, 196, 245, 252
Retamozo, Jesus   245
Reyes, Estephany   245
Riquett, Mary   252
Rodriguez-Aguilar, Roman   73, 216
Rodriguez-Aguilar, Román   88
Rojas-Arce, Jorge L.   129

Salais-Fierro, Tomás E.   225
Sanchez-Jimenez, Loraine   225
Saucedo Martínez, Jania Astrid   3
Saucedo-Martinez, Jania Astrid   177
Sierra, Laura   245

Triana, Karen Acosta   196

Urbieta, Mitchell Santiago Kelley   216
Uribe, Elí Gerardo Zorrilla   28

Vanegas, Jaider   245

Wu, Xuting   45

Xie, Hongcheng   109